MENTAL HEALTH AND LEARNING DISABILITY

David Carpenter
John Turnbull

Additional contributions from
Alan Kay

First edition 1991
Reprinted 1992 1993
Revised 1994
Second edition 1996
Reprinted 1996
Published by
Macmillan Magazines Ltd
Porters South, Crinan St
London N1 9XW

Companies and representatives throughout the world

Printed in Great Britain by
Barwell Colour Print Ltd
Midsomer Norton
Bath

ISBN 0-333-64683-5

Contents

Introduction

The purpose of this module

The *Mental Health and Learning Disability* module has been divided into two Parts — Part 1: Mental Health; Part 2: Learning Disability. Each part has been written by different authors: *Mental Health* by David Carpenter, and *Learning Disability* by Alan Kay, with contributions from John Turnbull. This highlights the fact that mental health and learning disability are two separate nursing specialisms dealing with very different client groups.

This module is one of the three specialist modules:

- *Care of the Mother and Newborn*
- *Community Health Care*
- *Mental Health and Learning Disability*

which form part of the Macmillan Open Learning/*Nursing Times* Open Learning Conversion Programme and is designed to be used in conjunction with the three core modules:

- *Professional Development*
- *Management*
- *Research.*

Each of the modules can also be used on its own for professional updating, or as a reference when a relevant experience arises.

The specialist modules can be studied at convenient times agreed between yourself, your tutor/counsellor and those organisations whose co-operation you need to further your experience in the case of each module.

The *Mental Health and Learning Disability* module and your related experience are not intended to turn you into a specialist mental health or learning disability nurse. The experience you gain will enable you to develop an understanding of the impact of mental illness and learning disability on the people concerned, and those who care for them, be they from the professional health services, the voluntary sector or the immediate family.

You will also have the opportunity to see the way in which the resources available to support and care for mentally ill people and those with a learning disability and their families are organised.

How to use this module

In order to register as a first-level nurse, the UKCC requires that your conversion programme includes a minimum of 60 hours on community health care and 150 hours each on the care of the mother and newborn and mental health and learning disability, including theory and experience.

When and how you gain your experience of mental health and/or learning disability will depend on your tutor/counsellor and the relevant nursing managers although we recommend that you work through Sections 1 and 2 of the *Community Health Care* module before you start on this specialist module because it contains essential information on demography and its relationship to the provision of care.

The material in the three specialist modules contains more work than the UKCC minimums specified above for first-level registration. However, you may find that by dovetailing some aspects of the project work, based on the community profile (see below), you can be working on more than one module at the same time. The student notes which accompany these modules give more guidance on planning and management of this work.

The community profile

Throughout the three modules, *Community Health Care*, *Care of the Mother and Newborn*, and *Mental Health and Learning Disability*, you will be asked to include in your community profile relevant information you obtain from carrying out some of the Activities you undertake.

Do not confuse the community profile with your personal profile. It is an entirely separate document.

The community profile will provide a record — a picture — of the community in which you and your clients live and work, in particular:

• The people who make up the community
• Their health and social and cultural needs
• The resources and services available to meet those needs.

If you live and work in a large urban area, your community profile may represent only a part of a larger community. However, if you live and work in a rural area, you may be able to develop a picture of a much larger section of the community, if not the entire community.

Whatever your practice setting or specialism, the community profile should become a very useful resource for you.

As the community profile grows it will enable you to demonstrate your developing knowledge and understanding of the community and your client/patient group. It will also offer a point of reference from which to illustrate the changes which occur, especially in resources and services, and your increasing ability to understand the possible effects of these changes on you and your clients/patients.

Building your community profile

Where do you keep it?
You may wish to keep your community profile in a section of your student pack binder. Alternatively, you may find it more convenient to keep it in a separate binder altogether.

How do you develop it?
You are free to develop the community profile as you wish, creating sections or categories which best meet your learning objectives.

However, one suggestion is that you divide it into the sections we described above, namely:

- The people — looking at the different cultural, religious and social groups, where and at what many of them work, how supportive they are of each other, and in particular those who make up your client group.

- The health, social and cultural needs of the community — again looking at your particular group, or the community as a whole.

- The resources and services available to meet those needs — for example, shopping, transport, leisure and sporting facilities and health, voluntary and social services.

You may decide to expand on these sections, sub-divide them, or create entirely different ones.

However you create it, the profile should give you the information you need to help you provide an appropriate service for your clients.

SYMBOLS

The following information will explain the symbols that accompany the Activities in this module.

The times given for Activities are approximate only and are intended to reflect the actual time spent with an individual or reading information. They also include the time spent making notes. The time it takes to locate the people or information you need will undoubtedly vary enormously and would, therefore, be impossible to estimate.

Your diary is your own private record of your course work. Use it to make notes of your own ideas and opinions about the work you are doing. You will find it particularly helpful to jot down answers to those Activities with the diary symbol, as they may be used as the basis for discussion.

Activities accompanied by this sign are reflective Activities, which ask you to think about a particular point in the text before reading on. You may decide that it would be useful to record these in your diary as well.

Some of the Activities ask you to do practical things, which you may not be able to complete during the period you are working on a particular section. If this is the case, you should use your programme planner to record dates when you will be able to carry them out.

Some of the Activities encourage you to include the material you gather in your community profile. This is designed to help you record your developing knowledge of the community and is therefore a key tool in the work you do for this part of the programme. (See the notes on pages 4 and 5 about building a community profile.)

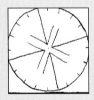

At the end of each Section of the module we will provide a Focus Activity, which is intended to draw together the ideas and situations you have been exploring, and to relate them to your own experience and locality. There will almost certainly be some written work in the Focus Activity and it may also involve research, review or discussion.

1. What is mental health?

Introduction

The health of everyone is affected by physical, psychological and social factors and nursing care is unlikely to be effective unless it encompasses the needs of the whole person. You may never have contemplated nursing mentally ill people, although in planning care in other contexts it is likely that you have identified problems relating to mental health as well as physical health. There are, of course, clients who are primarily mentally ill and those who are primarily physically ill, but nurses should aim always to practise holistically. All nurses therefore need some mental health knowledge and experience in order to:

- Plan care and practise holistically and not treat the client as just a body in which a disease exists
- Care for a mentally ill person who is receiving treatment for another aspect of his/her health.

You will already have some experience of dealing with mental health issues, because you will have been involved in assessing and planning those aspects of psychosocial care which are included in every client's care plan. You may not have seen these issues as directly relating to mental health, but, as we shall see in this Section, for most general nurses it is the psychosocial aspects of care which are most important in determining the level of mental health of the client.

Let us start by thinking about these aspects of your practice.

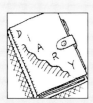

ACTIVITY 1
10-15 mins
Think about three clients for whom you are currently caring. Make some notes in your diary on:

- **Psychosocial aspects of their care which have already been planned**

- **How their psychosocial needs were identified, and by whom.**

While a client's physical care needs can usually be assessed and planned using criteria which are fairly *objective*, that is, described and understood by everyone in more or less the same way, his/her psychosocial needs have to be looked at from a completely different standpoint. Assessment of the psychosocial needs of the individual is a subjective process, in which the values, attitudes and beliefs of the person making the assessment are as much a part of the process as those of the client.

ACTIVITY 2
20-30 mins
Think again about the three clients you considered in Activity 1:

• Describe them in as many ways as you can that are not based on their symptoms or diagnosed illness. Your descriptions could include such things as social ties, age, or work environment (for example, a 38-year-old unemployed father of three school-age children who was admitted as an emergency last night)

• Now use these descriptions to determine the needs and problems which you think those clients have which might be psychosocially based

• Compare your conclusions with those laid down in the original care plans, and make notes in your diary of any differences you find.

In this Activity, you have begun to explore some of the issues relating to how psychosocial needs and mental health problems can be defined. In this first Section of the Mental Health module, we discuss these issues further, by examining some of the concepts on which our view of mental health is based.

In the second Section, we look at the role of the nurse in caring for clients who have mental health problems, and consider the importance of being aware of your own values, attitudes and beliefs about mental illness.

We then go on to look at some of the skills you may need to develop to provide care for any client who is experiencing psychosocial or mental health problems.

The final Section of the Mental Health module explores some wider issues about the best way to provide care in this area.

Health and mental health

An individual's state of health is usually a subjective matter, based on that individual's view of what health is and what illness is. To illustrate this let us take the example of people with diabetes. According to objective, scientific criteria, diabetes is a serious disorder if not properly managed. However, the way in which those who have this condition see their general state of health will vary enormously, depending on their personal views of health and illness. People with diabetes whose condition is stable might see themselves as completely healthy if they felt that it did not affect their life to any great extent. On the other hand, if they felt that the measures they had to take to keep their condition stable did affect certain important areas of their life (such as being able to eat out), then they might consider that they were not completely healthy.

When it comes to mental health, however, definitions are much less clear-cut. As we saw above, assessments about a person's mental health must always be subjective, and because of this, there is an enormous amount of controversy about what mental health and mental illness are. Added to this is the fact that people who, by any definition, are mentally ill, often see themselves as quite the reverse.

What is health?

The most frequently quoted definition of health is that given by the World Health Organisation[1]:

❝ Health is a state of complete physical, mental, and social well-being, and not merely the absence of disease or infirmity ❞.

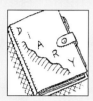

ACTIVITY 3
3-5 mins
Write a sentence describing what you consider to be a state of 'complete mental well-being'.

How often do you think it is possible to reach this state?

We can only guess at what you wrote here — different people will have their own ideas about what constitutes 'well-being'. You might, for example, have written 'absence of worry', or 'lack of anxiety', or you might have been more descriptive, perhaps mentioning feelings of inner peace, or 'being at one with the world'.

We would be surprised if you said it was never possible to achieve this state completely. However, you may have said that it is not easy to maintain a state of complete mental well-being for very long — the pressures, demands and worries of everyday life tend to act against this.

You may also have found that a state of mental well-being is not easy to assess. Fears, worries and stress, for example, can affect mental well-being but, as we saw above, most people would not consider themselves to be mentally unhealthy merely because they have a few worries. There would be a problem only if the worries were so preoccupying that these people were unable to lead their lives as they would wish. So mental health might be a matter of people feeling in control of their own lives.

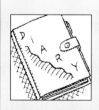

ACTIVITY 4
5-10 mins
What does 'being in control of your life' mean to you? Make some notes in your diary.

Once again, your response to this Activity will depend on your own views and beliefs. Some people believe that they should be in control of all aspects of their life, and blame themselves if things go wrong. Others believe that everything in life is controlled by fate, or by God, and feel that they themselves have very little influence on the course of their lives. You may find it interesting to discuss this question with other people in your life and see how views can vary.

Most people experience occasions when they feel as though they no longer have as much control over their life as usual. For example, if they are seriously ill it is likely that they will be unable to do all the things that they would wish — they lose control, and this is frightening.

We could say, then, that:

Mental Health is a state of well-being resulting from a feeling of being in control over one's own life.

If we accept this definition, we can see that we all have mental health problems from time to time. Even a common cold can interfere with day-to-day control over our own life. It is well known that influenza is a common cause of depression and, although theories attempting to account for this are complex, loss of personal control, feelings of vulnerability and recognition of the fact that we have no means of avoiding the effect of a simple virus all provide part of the explanation.

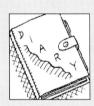

ACTIVITY 5
30 mins
Try to recall the last time that you felt you were not in control of your own life.

- What caused your loss of control?

- What did you feel like? Write down some of the feelings.

- Ask a friend or relative who recalls your behaviour to explain the changes which occurred. Write a brief account.

- How did you regain control? Write down the circumstances (people, things or events) which helped you.

  Record your answers in your diary.

You can probably see that you yourself have experienced some problems which affected your mental well-being. The events you described in answer to the previous Activity would certainly represent a deviation from the WHO definition of 'a state of complete mental well-being'. Most of us experience these sorts of problem from time to time, and most of us find ways of dealing with them without too much long-term disadvantage to our physical or social well-being.

So if 'complete mental well-being' is a state which most of us seldom achieve, when does a mental health problem become a condition requiring professional intervention?

Normality and abnormality
Many people, when questioned, will admit that they have felt the urge, at one time or another, to jump off a tall building or into the path of an oncoming train. These feelings are fairly common, and are difficult

to explain, since many of the people who experience them have no immediate threat to their mental well-being at all. Even if we do feel a bit depressed, or overburdened with life's problems, most of us still would not succumb to the urge to end our life.

So we can see that even if we lose control over certain aspects of our lives, and may feel like jumping off a high building or murdering the kids, we do not actually do it. Our thought processes ensure that feelings such as these are not translated into action. We could therefore add a rider to our previous definition of mental health so that it reads:

Mental Health is a state of well-being resulting from a feeling of being in control over one's life. Control over normal feelings is maintained by rational thought processes.

So, using this above definition, *feeling* like jumping off a high building or murdering the kids could be regarded as fairly 'normal', but actually *doing* them is 'abnormal'.

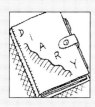

ACTIVITY 6
5-10 mins
Without looking at a dictionary, write down your own definitions of 'normal' and 'abnormal'.

Most definitions of normality refer to something which conforms to commonly-agreed standards or levels. This is fine when we talk about an X-ray, or the results of a biopsy, for example. The standards of 'normality' in these cases are based on scientific research which gives us a measure of what we might expect to see in a healthy body, and 'abnormal' is a measure which anyone can judge against this standard.

'Abnormality' in this context is an *objective* measure — something which is not a matter of opinion, but which can be judged in the same way by everyone, against a standard which everyone understands.

In other areas, however, the notion of commonly-agreed standards is much less straightforward. Even some kinds of physical illness, which can be diagnosed according to standards agreed by the medical profession as a condition which deviates from the standard of a 'healthy body', may not be regarded in the same way by the person who is held to be 'suffering' from it. Diabetes is a good example of this. As we saw earlier, this is a serious disorder if it is not managed properly. However, most people with diabetes do not regard themselves as 'abnormal' simply because they have diabetes, and do, indeed, live perfectly 'normal' lives.

We can see from this that the concept of 'normality' can be based on the opinions of individual people even when there are technical standards by which 'normality' can be measured. These *subjective* opinions are based on the values, attitudes and beliefs of each individual, and can be shaped by a whole range of factors, such as their background and personal history.

Sedgwick[2] provides another example of this. He describes a South

American Indian tribe where those suffering from the disease dyschromic spirochetosis, in which coloured spots appear on the skin, are considered normal, while those who would be described objectively as 'healthy', that is, not having the disease, are regarded as abnormal, and are excluded from marriage.

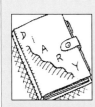

ACTIVITY 7
20 mins
Would you use the term 'abnormal' for any of the clients for whom you are caring?

Explan why you
• would use the term
• would not use the term.

Note down your thoughts in your diary.

It is doubtful whether you would describe any of your clients as 'abnormal' just because they are physically unhealthy. Being unhealthy does not mean being abnormal. Despite this, people with comparatively minor mental health problems are often referred to as abnormal. Such people are certainly not abnormal and it is doubtful whether minor changes in behaviour can really be defined as abnormal.

How did you feel about giving the label 'abnormal' to any of your clients? Describing people and their behaviour in this way is a subjective *value judgement*, based on our own values, attitudes and beliefs. As such, defining a person as 'abnormal' reflects our own perception of what is normal.

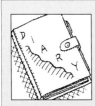

ACTIVITY 8
15-20 mins
Reflect on your answer to Activity 7 above. What idea of normality did you have in mind when deciding what your answer would be?

Make some notes in your diary.

This question is at the heart of one of the great debates in mental health — when does a mental health problem which would generally be considered 'normal' become mental illness? Does mental illness exist, or is it something which is *socially constructed*, created by society to explain behaviour which does not conform to that which is socially acceptable?

Mental health and disease: the debates

It is clear that some people suffer from serious impairments of mental health such that there is little doubt that they are mentally ill. But how do we describe this illness? Consider the following description of schizophrenia, which is a serious mental illness:

•A large group of disorders, usually of psychotic proportion, manifested by characteristic disturbances of language and communication, thought, perception, affect and behaviour which lasts longer than six months. Thought disturbances are marked by alterations of concept formation that may lead to misinterpretation of reality, misperceptions and sometimes to delusions and hallucinations. Mood changes include ambivalence, blunting, inappropriateness, and loss of empathy with others. Behaviour may be withdrawn, aggressive and bizarre'[3].

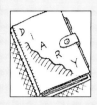

ACTIVITY 9
30 mins
Look up any unfamiliar words that appear in this description and then rewrite it in your diary in your own words, so that you are easily able to understand it.

Now that you have a more accessible description, it is possible to consider mental illness in more detail. Do the words used in the description above actually describe an objective state of affairs or is it a subjective judgement, that is, an expression of approval or disapproval based on concepts of 'normality'?

Szasz[4], a well-known anti-psychiatrist, claims that there is no such thing as mental illness. He believes there are some people who have what he calls 'problems in living' (for example, homelessness, isolation, criminal activity), and that it suits society to give such people a label. Schizophrenia is merely one label for the problems some people have in social adjustment. It is not a disease as we normally understand the term but a fabrication designed to medicalise what should properly be understood as social deviation.

Szasz's views are vigorously contested by most members of the medical profession. However, the description given above is typical of the way schizophrenia has conventionally been described by the medical profession, even though it was suggested that there may be a physical cause of the disease — an excess of the neuro-transmitter dopamine.

It is also interesting to note that, in diagnosing mental illness, the dividing line between eccentricity and insanity is often determined by social factors, so that 'nice' people (including our own friends and relatives) are eccentric, or have 'nervous breakdowns', while more offensive descriptions, such as 'mad' or 'insane', are reserved for others.

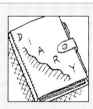

ACTIVITY 10
30 mins
Look again at the description of schizophrenia which begins on page 12.

- Is it objective; that is, does it refer to a state of affairs which would be the case regardless of whether there was someone else to observe it, or is it subjective, essentially a collection of statements of approval or disapproval?

- Imagine that you are a neighbour of a person who manifests these symptoms. What problems might you experience in relating with this person? What problems might the person have in relating with you?

Note down your responses in your diary.

You may have concluded from this Activity that the boundaries of mental illness are potentially very wide. They will depend largely upon what is agreed to be normal behaviour by the majority of people in society. Once a person's behaviour has been recognised as 'abnormal', it is then a short step to the formation of a value-laden description of that person's condition, such as the one above. This may then be swiftly followed by the alienation of that person from 'normal' life.

Having said this, we do not wish to suggest that mental disease does not exist, nor that it is not the concern of medicine. Nor do we wish to suggest that mental health is alone in using subjective judgements, as the example we gave earlier of the Indians with the skin disease showed.

What we are emphasising, however, is that because most medical diagnoses of mental illness are, in fact, expressed in subjective terms, the implication for nurses who care for those with mental illness is therefore that the *attitudes* of the carers are as important as their skills.

It is interesting to note that the issues discussed in this Section are clear to many clients:

"Suggesting someone is ill is better than suggesting they are bad, as they used to do. However, this is not an illness like measles, a broken leg or diabetes, and society knows this" [5].

In the next Section, we ask you to explore some of your own values, attitudes and beliefs about people with mental illness, and consider why it is important to be aware of these when caring for such people.

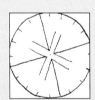

FOCUS
1 hour
Look back to your answers to Activities 1 and 2 at the beginning of this section. Read through the descriptions you wrote of each of the three clients, and the psychosocial needs you identified, and make a note of any value judgements they contain.

When you have done this, try to describe each of the three clients as they might see themselves. How many value judgements does the description include now?

What are the major differences between the descriptions?

2. The importance of self-awareness

This Section explores the issue of self-awareness and the preparation of self for effective clinical intervention. Bond[1], Brill[2] and Burnard[3] examine these issues in greater detail.

The role of the nurse in mental health care

At the end of the previous Section, we suggested that nurses and anyone else connected with a client with mental health problems have a duty to attempt to understand the client, and to be aware of their own attitudes to the client's condition.

So how important is this factor in the role of the mental health nurse?

Although it is clear that the mental health nurse is to some extent concerned with practical, physical aspects of care, we could argue that this part of the nurse's work is not the most significant. In addition to *doing* certain things, all nurses are also required to *be* certain things; for example, understanding, patient, supportive, comforting.

In caring for clients with mental health problems, these 'being' aspects of the nurses' role are often more important than the 'doing' aspects.

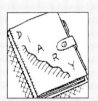

ACTIVITY 1
10-15 mins
Think about the 'being' aspects of your own role. What do you think your clients need you to be? What difficulties do you have in meeting those needs?

Make some notes in your diary.

The 'being' aspect of the nurse's role demands that we understand both what it is clients want and how we ourselves respond to that need. This requires that we understand not only our clients, but also ourselves: that we are aware of how we relate and respond to them and their condition. When dealing with clients with mental health problems, this is even more necessary, because, as we saw in the previous Section, the definition of the illness itself is usually subjective, based on individual values, attitudes and beliefs.

The key to this understanding is an awareness of ourselves, our own values, attitudes and beliefs: 'where we are coming from', what 'makes us tick', what our 'hang-ups' are.

Why do we need to be more self-aware?

We have already seen that describing a person as having a mental health problem is, in essence, a value judgement. You have no thermometers or other devices to make an objective assessment of a client's mental health status. The only measure available to you as a nurse in assessing the nature of a client's mental health problem is you yourself.

It is therefore important that your idea of 'self' is well calibrated; that is, that you understand the measures you are using when you make judgements about other people.

To illustrate this, you might consider the times when you get angry. If you have a fairly high level of self-awareness, you will have a good idea of what sorts of people, things or situations tend to make you angry.

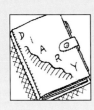

ACTIVITY 2
5-10 mins
Try and describe some of the people, things or situations which almost always have the effect of making you angry.

Recognising the effects of the things that make you angry might also lead you to realise that when you *do* get angry, your anger might be out of proportion to the situation which has provoked it. If you understand that this is a feature of 'you', that is, if you are aware of this aspect of self, you are less likely to fall into the trap of attributing whatever it was that provoked your anger to the thing or individual concerned.

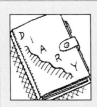

ACTIVITY 3
5-10 mins
Reflect on your answers to Activity 2 above. Can you think of any situations when your anger was out of proportion to the situation? If so, describe what happened, and suggest reasons.

Understanding where your anger comes from gives you a scale, or measure, against which you can judge any angry reactions you feel in the future. This is an example of how increased self-awareness gives you a greater understanding of how you react with other people and situations.

Self-awareness in nurse-client interaction

Being aware of how you react to a whole range of different situations is at the heart of creating the effective nurse-client relationships which are so important in mental health nursing. We now explore some issues of self-awareness which can occur fairly commonly in situations where a nurse uses her 'self' as therapy, that is, where she is *being* something to help the client, rather than *doing* something to help the client.

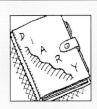

ACTIVITY 4
20 mins
What do you mean when you find yourself saying things such as: 'I don't know whether it is her or me but...'

Write one or two paragraphs in your diary, trying to explain the issues involved.

You might have suggested that the problem is simply a difficulty in understanding another person's perspective: you view something in a particular way while the other person sees it entirely differently. Who is right?

We are often tempted to believe that we are right and the other person is wrong. Sometimes we are so sure of our own opinions that we lose sight of the possibility that when we describe another person or a particular situation we are likely to colour the description according to our own beliefs. In fact, in an extreme case, when we say something about someone else we might be revealing more about ourselves than about them.

This attributing another person with behaviour which is actually your own is called *projection*. The example we gave above, about things or situations that make you angry, is another example of projection: you might have projected intense feelings of anger onto someone who had not done anything to deserve them. In doing this, you were saying something about yourself, and your reactions to certain things, rather than about the individual concerned.

Understanding how the process of projection works may help you to recognise it in yourself and others.

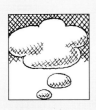

ACTIVITY 5
20 mins
Think of someone about whom you have particularly strong feelings. Try to analyse your view critically. Is the person really as you describe, or is there the possibility that you might be saying something about yourself?

This Activity might have caused you to question some of the opinions you have held so far about the other person. If you have not, just think about the last time you complained about how opinionated another person was. Ask yourself how you described that person. Was it really in a non-opinionated way?

Increased self-awareness will help you to ensure that when you are describing another person you are really talking about the person and not about yourself. For example, if you are convinced that someone else does not like you, are you really sure that it is not *you* who does not like you?

ACTIVITY 6
2 hours
Projection is more common than most people realise. One way you could practise recognising it is to think about the ways in which some of the more stereotyped characters in television soap operas describe each other.

Next time you watch a 'soap', look out for some of the behaviours we have described above, such as people believing they are always right, people colouring descriptions of others with their own views, and saying something about someone else when they are really describing themselves.

Once you have practised on this 'artificial' situation, you can use what you have observed to recognise examples of projection in yourself and in others at work and in your everyday life.

Another example of when the 'ownership' of feelings can get confused is when you come home feeling 'awful' but you do not know why. It is possible that the feelings you have are not really yours. Nurses can easily become 'sponges', and soak up other people's feelings. Have you ever spoken to another person who is very worried, but at the end of the conversation although that person feels much better you feel much worse? This is called *introjection*. While such a situation might help the other person in the short term, no nurse can continue to absorb other people's problems in this way.

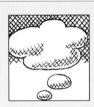

ACTIVITY 7
20 mins
Think of the last time you came home feeling 'awful'. Try to identify whether those feelings really belonged to you or whether there was a chance that you had absorbed another person's problems.

Recognising the existence of this process and whether or not it happens to you could help to avert a potential personal disaster and, moreover, will ensure that you move beyond merely absorbing other people's problems to helping them solve them.

A third phenomenon in nursing is *transference*.

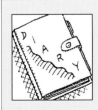

ACTIVITY 8
10-15 mins
Can you think of an occasion when a client had particularly strong feelings for you?

Describe what happened, and how you responded to it.

This type of situation is not unusual; after all, many clients are extremely grateful for the care they receive. Sometimes, however, the feelings extend beyond this level. It is possible for a client to have feelings towards a nurse which are actually not directed at the nurse herself but at another person represented by the nurse. For example, the nurse may represent a parent who has always offered security and care, or a partner or a friend in whom the client can confide.

This process, in which the client's feelings for one person are transferred to another, is called *transference*. Being aware of how this situation can arise, and how you respond to it, can help you to handle it appropriately.

Attitudes and prejudices

Increased self-awareness can also help you to identify your own particular attitudes and prejudices. Do you hold any views which might affect the quality of care you offer? 'No!' you may reply, and this would not be surprising, since most of us believe what are really prejudices to be statements of fact.

For example, it is common to claim that smokers waste health-care resources; they are frequently seen as second-class clients. No one is suggesting that smoking is a good thing nor that it should not be discouraged, but should smokers be rejected (even covertly) because they waste resources? The facts of this issue are actually quite surprising! Smokers actually save resources because they are very likely to die before they take advantage of many of the health services; moreover, smokers contribute large sums of money in taxation.

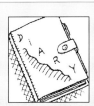

ACTIVITY 9
20 mins
There is little doubt that some clients are more popular than others, and this has been well described by Stockwell[4].

- What sorts of clients are most popular with you?

- Try to be honest and make a list of types of clients in order of their popularity with you. Can you spot any prejudices? Discuss your list with a colleague.

- Make comments in your diary.

Do you still believe that you have no particular prejudices? Did your colleague help you to highlight any attitudes of which you were not aware?

Our attitudes and prejudices can also affect the care we provide even before we meet a client.

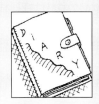

ACTIVITY 10
10-15 mins
Note down in you diary any advantages and disadvantages of receiving information about clients before you meet them?

On the positive side, information might help you to prepare for the clients, either by giving you an insight into particular needs, or by allowing you to reflect on your attitudes to the information you have received.

On the negative side, however, the information you receive may colour your attitude before you have even met the person. It is important to be aware of the tendency to accept information provided by others which might actually be saying more about them than about the person to whom it refers. We must be able to distinguish between the expression of the attitudes of others and the genuine recording of facts. Of course, there is nothing wrong with recording personal opinions and beliefs but they should be identified as such so that the reader can be absolutely clear about their origins.

Such information might also connect with some of your own feelings, which might prevent you from working effectively with the client. For example, a nurse who has been recently bereaved might find it difficult to work with a client who has a problem connected with grief.

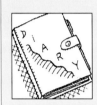

ACTIVITY 11
15 mins
Think of an occasion when your own feelings might have affected your interactions with a client.

Make notes in your diary.

Being aware of any tendencies towards projection or introjection in yourself, knowing when you are the object of transference and being able to recognise your own attitudes and prejudices, will help you to gain self-awareness which, in turn, will help you to understand other people better.

The use of 'self' as therapy
Once you have a greater degree of self-awareness, it is possible to use the 'self' therapeutically. The higher your level of self-awareness, the more likely it is that you will be able to 'be' what it is that your clients need you to be.

At the end of the first Section, we asked you to describe three of your clients as *they would describe themselves*. The ability to feel as if we were another person is called *empathy*. Rogers[5] describes empathy as the ability to enter the world of another as if it were your own.

Empathy is an important tool in understanding a client's feelings, but it can only be really effective if the nurse can continue to distinguish between the two worlds. This can be quite difficult if the nurse is not aware of which feelings are her own and which belong to the client.

Empathising with another person is a way of managing your own feelings to benefit another person. *Sympathy*, on the other hand, is an expression of your feelings.

Sympathy is not usually a helpful therapeutic tool. People are often sympathetic simply because it makes *them* feel better, perhaps in that they have been able to give some sort of response to a problem they cannot really do very much about. That is not to say that sympathy is not offered with the best intentions, but that it does very little to help a nurse *understand* another person's feelings.

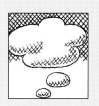

ACTIVITY 12
5-10 mins
Think about the last time you offered sympathy to a client? Were you really trying to cope with your own feelings about the situation rather than understand those of the client?

Sometimes, we express sympathy by recounting a personal experience which has aspects in common with the client's problem, for example, 'When I had my operation. . .' or 'When someone close to me died. . .' *Self-disclosure* such as this can be effective in providing therapy, provided it is based on an understanding of how the client will receive the information (that is, based on an empathetic understanding of how the client will react) rather than simply as an illustration of how someone else coped (that is, look how well I coped, why can't you?). It is also important to ensure that the client is not being used as a listener to the nurse's own problems.

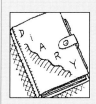

ACTIVITY 13
30 mins
Read the following short case study and make some brief notes in your diary on the client, and any problems you might anticipate if you were the nurse in the description.

> Gladys Miles, a 58-year-old single woman, was referred for radical mastectomy following positive diagnosis of carcinoma. She believed strongly that the consequent disfigurement would be so severe that the treatment would be best avoided. A nurse was asked to talk with Gladys to help her make an informed choice.

It is likely that the nurse's own life experiences, including personal contacts with friends or relatives who have been in a similar position to Gladys, would have a bearing on the help offered to Gladys. It is also possible that the nurse would have particular personal fears about this or related illnesses and these fears would substantially affect how the client was helped unless the nurse was aware of the fears and was able to compensate for them. If Gladys resolved not to have the treatment, the nurse's feelings could be particularly intense.

Good communication is the key to effective nurse–client interaction. In the example above, if the nurse was unable to overcome personal feelings in order to communicate openly with Gladys, it would be difficult to help Gladys make an informed choice.

In the next Section, we will be exploring in more detail some important communication skills, but we end this Section by looking at your own abilities as a communicator.

What sort of communicator are you?

Purposeful verbal and non-verbal communication is an important part of psychosocial nursing care. As we saw at the start of this Section, in mental health nursing the personal qualities of the nurse are part of the treatment. In this context, an awareness of how you communicate is therefore a necessary pre-requisite of effective care in mental health.

The following is an exercise in non-verbal communication: how well do you communicate if you do not actually say anything?

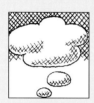

ACTIVITY 14
30 mins
This task could be undertaken alone with the use of a mirror, but it is far more effective if you can get a friend to work with you.

Make a list of emotions, for example anger, sadness, happiness, joy, anxiety, perplexity. Mime the facial expressions of these emotions to a friend, or, if you are alone, in front of a mirror.

Do your expressions vary sufficiently or could they be misleading? What are the potential dangers of misleading facial expressions (for example, some people frown when they are puzzled)?

If you can find some obliging friends, you can use the exercise to help you become more skilled in recognising emotional expressions. Take it in turns to mime the emotions and see whether it is possible to identify the emotion portrayed.

Non-verbal communication (particularly in the form of facial expression) often tells the truth, whereas verbal communication can be controlled to the extent that it can readily mislead. It is therefore imperative that nurses are aware of the messages they convey non-verbally, and, more important, that they are able to recognise their clients' messages.

For example, clients might not necessarily express fears and other emotions verbally, but their facial expression may reveal much about what they are feeling. The skilled nurse will use a wide range of perceptual ability in order to anticipate the needs and wishes of clients.

You may have had the very comfortable experience of communicating with another person who is really able to understand you. This skill is achieved by heightened awareness of self and others, and can be practised using the following Activity.

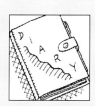

ACTIVITY 15
30 mins
Look for non-verbal communication in others — perhaps on public transport or in some other public place.

Look for facial expressions. What do you think they convey? Look at body posture as well. What do you think the person is feeling? More important, ask a friend or colleague what your facial expressions and body postures convey to others.

Note down your observations in your diary.

This type of activity can increase your powers of observation of other people's non-verbal communication, and also develop an awareness of your own personal style. Do you show emotion readily? Do you conceal what you are thinking so that others think you have few emotions?

Verbal communication can be analysed in a similar way. Verbal communication is not just about what is said, but is also about how it is said. It can also just as easily be about what is not said. A person who talks a lot is not necessarily someone who has a lot to say! For example, a client might talk a great deal largely because of deep anxiety, so imagine the verbal chaos that would ensue if the nurse also kept talking because of feeling anxious! The importance of silence will be considered later. Meanwhile, try to improve your verbal communication by working through the following Activity.

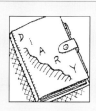

ACTIVITY 16
1 hour
Now that you have worked through this Section on self-awareness, describe the following to some friends while sitting on your hands:

- A fountain
- Cornflakes
- The weather.

When you have thought about your own views on how you communicate, ask your friends how successful your descriptions seemed to them and compare your answers with theirs. This will help you to discover your strongest form of communication, both from the point of view of conveying information as well as receiving it.

Ask yourself if your descriptions show that you usually choose your words wisely. Do you describe things as you see them, as you hear them or as you feel them?

Individuals tend to have different preferences in communication, so knowing your own preferences can help you discover a lot about yourself. Your increased awareness of communication preferences should also help you to communicate more effectively with patients by using language which respects their preferences.

Record your findings in your diary.

This Section has focused on the importance of self-awareness in mental health nursing. Thinking about all the issues that have been raised will help to raise your own level of self-awareness in the context of how you relate to your clients.

For the Focus Activity, we would like you to take the opportunity to indulge in some reflection about your general state of self-awareness.

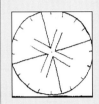

FOCUS
45-60 mins
Spend about 10 minutes thinking about and writing down the things you are aware of around you, such as sounds, smells, feelings and sights; as you do so also note down any memories prompted by those sensations.

Preface each sentence with a phrase such as 'Now', 'At this minute', (for example, 'Now I am aware of cars passing').

After 10 minutes, study your list and count:

• The number of times you stayed in the present
• The number of times you thought of future events
• The number of times you recalled past events.

Did you dwell in the future (Now I am wondering what to cook for dinner) or the past (Now I am thinking about the row I had at work) or were you alert to what it is possible to be aware of in the here and now?

Look at your list again. Note down whether the things of which you were aware were mainly external (what was going on outside the room, or in the world at large), whether you were primarily aware of things that were happening to you physically (tired, headache, itch, hunger), or whether you focused on things which were happening to you emotionally (bored, angry, alert, interested).

If you found that you focused more on some areas than others, make some notes in your diary on the steps you could take to ensure that you develop a more balanced self-awareness.

3. Mental health nursing skills

This Section introduces some of the specific skills and techniques which are useful in providing psychosocial care. It is important to remember, however, that simply using the techniques makes one only a technician. Nursing should extend beyond this to include a genuine therapeutic use of self, as we saw in the previous Section, by recognising that the relationship between nurse and client plays a key role in overall treatment and care.

In Section 2, you were asked the question: 'What sort of communicator are you?' The answers you gave to the Activities related to that question will have given you some insight into your strengths as a communicator, and may also have indicated areas where you might need to develop communication skills. Bear these in mind as you work through this Section.

Listening

Listening is a necessary and integral part of any communication, and care should always be planned on the basis of a partnership, with each partner respecting the other and taking the time to listen to the other.

On occasions, nurses can be so concerned with talking to clients that they can easily forget the need to listen. One of the reasons for behaving like this might be the nurse's own anxiety. This anxiety could be caused by the nurse sincerely wishing to be helpful but actually not being sure how to be.

Active listening requires you to concentrate on what the other person is saying and on how it is being said. It also requires you to be aware of your own body posture and other non-verbal behaviour, so that you are clear about the messages you are sending back to the person to whom you are listening.

The following Activity will help you discover how effective your listening skills are.

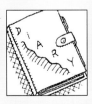

ACTIVITY 1
20-30 mins
Ask a friend to talk for five minutes about family or friends whom you do not know. You may ask questions to clarify anything that is not clear to you. After five minutes stop and recount the information to your friend and ask whether you missed anything out.

A third person may act as an observer and give feedback on your ability to listen actively.

Cont...

... cont

- **What did you forget?**

- **How much did you remember?**

- **Did you find yourself being distracted by comparisons with your own friends and family or were you really able to maintain a constant interest in the descriptions given by your friend?**

Keep a record in your diary.

The difference between listening and hearing

Listening is not the same as hearing. We can all easily hear what we want to hear, but when we listen we really discover things about other people. Consider the following case study:

'You seem really busy today, Nurse,' said Mrs Brown, an elderly lady with diabetes who was due to have a below-knee amputation the following day.

'Yes, I am. The operation list is so long and as usual we are very short staffed. It's this bug you know; half the nurses seem to have been struck down by it. You are looking good today, is that a new nightie? I expect your grandchildren will be in later — the little lad is lovely, isn't he? Oh, there's Mrs Jones calling again. I expect her water jug is empty. Nice to talk to you, I will be back later. We'll have a chat about tomorrow. You're not too worried, are you?'

The nurse immediately went to the aid of Mrs Jones.

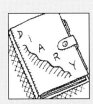

ACTIVITY 2
5-10 mins
If the nurse in the description above had listened to Mrs Brown, do you think that the 'conversation' would have been different?

- **What do you think Mrs Brown might really have been saying?**

- **Why do you think the nurse behaved as she did?**

Make some notes in your diary.

Without more detail, we cannot really make a judgement here. However, you might have suggested that Mrs Brown was really asking for attention herself, and was making a rather oblique reference to the fact that she was anxious about tomorrow, but no one seemed to have time to talk to her.

The nurse may genuinely have failed to pick up on this because she did not really listen to what Mrs Brown was saying. For whatever reason, she may not have wanted to get involved in such a discussion at that time, so her action may have been an avoidance tactic.

By thinking about such points, the huge difference between listening and hearing should become evident. The example also provides a good case of an anxious nurse who may be worried about giving the client an opportunity to talk because of feeling unable to help.

Starting a conversation with a client

Starting a conversation with a person is not always easy. Comments about the weather rarely lead to a mutually rewarding conversation and topics such as politics are probably best avoided. It is clear that the first few words are vitally important in setting the scene for future interactions. The following task will help you to gain some insights into your current practice.

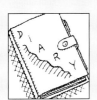

ACTIVITY 3
30 mins
Write down in your diary a list of the sorts of things you tend to say to clients when you first meet them or after you have not seen them for a few days.

Now look closely at your list. Have you tended to ask questions? Were they open, allowing the clients to expand and talk about themselves and their problems, or were they closed questions providing for 'Yes' or 'No' answers only?

Open questions allow more scope and give the client responsibilities and some control within the interaction. Examples of such 'broad openings' include: 'How have you been since we last met?' (Compare this with 'Have you been well since we last met?').

Of course, just asking a person how he/she has been since you last met is not in itself sufficient. There is no point in a nurse asking a client a question unless the nurse is really interested in the answer and cares about the client, otherwise the question is merely rhetorical. The client is not required to answer and therefore no further interaction will follow.

Caring about ...

'You should not get emotionally involved with clients' is a much-stated maxim. It is often suggested that involvement is necessarily unprofessional. Professional nurses simply do not feel sad when a client is told that she is terminally ill, for example. There is some truth in this. After all, inappropriate involvement might well be unprofessional or it might result in nurses not being able to be helpful, as their emotion could block any ability to help. On the other hand, how can nurses truly be said to care unless they are *involved* with the client? The key, of course, is *appropriate involvement*. Professional caring entails managed emotional involvement.

What is professional caring? The following case will be helpful in understanding the reasons why the nurse should care about the client.

John Smithson was admitted to a medical ward following a serious overdose of drugs. He said that his life was not worth living since his wife had died: his only son had been killed in a road traffic accident and he had no other relatives. His life was empty, he said, and he had no particular interests and nothing that could be conceived as making his life worth living.

The nurse who was John's key worker felt very uncomfortable. Ideally, she would have liked to find arguments to convince him that his life was worth living but, at best, she could find only very feeble suggestions such as 'I am sure that people would miss you. Your neighbours have sent you a get well card, so they must be concerned'.

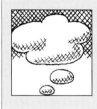

ACTIVITY 4
30 mins
Have you ever nursed someone like John? Can you think of any way John's nurse could stop him making a further attempt on his life?

It is very likely that John would feel very differently about the value of his life if someone else mattered to him or if he mattered to someone else. If the nurse could really show John that she cared about him — in other words, that it would matter to her if he were to die — it is at least possible that John's life might be saved. Sadly, there is often a tendency for nurses to show quite the opposite response (that is, to think that John matters less than other clients because he has caused his own problems). Moreover, some nurses believe that if John is treated very kindly, he will be more likely to attempt suicide again. You have probably heard people calling John's sort of behaviour 'attention seeking', implying that it should be ignored or even punished. However, if John is treated in this way he will be more likely to attempt suicide again, because his thoughts that his life is not worth living will have been confirmed.

Some nurses may hold the view that caring about John will do no good in the long run because as soon as he is discharged from hospital he will be back to square one and will attempt suicide again. This is not the sort of 'caring about' that we mean, as it only creates a dependence which will do more harm than good.

At the heart of John's problems is probably a lack of self-esteem, of self-worth. It is not so much a case of his *life* not being worth living as *his* life not being worth living. These are two fundamentally different situations. There is nothing, in the long term, that any nurse can do to *make* John's life worth living, but there is much that can be done to raise his self-esteem so that he is able to *feel* that his life is worth living. If John has the experience of being cared about, it will help him to realise that he is worth caring about. This realisation could lead to a long-term benefit, and is the aim of professional caring. In extreme cases like John's, it could be life-saving.

Allowing silence

Allowing silence is a skill in itself and is an example of what is often an anxiety-provoking situation for the nurse. It is sometimes difficult to assess whether the silence is beneficial to the client or not.

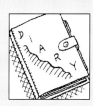

ACTIVITY 5
30 mins
Think back to a time when there was a period of silence during your involvement with a client and ask yourself the following questions:

- How long did the silence actually last?

- How long did you feel that it lasted?

- Who broke the silence, you or the client?

- How was the silence broken?

- Did the silence appear natural? Did it appear awkward? Did it follow on from what the client was previously saying or was the subject changed?

- Was the silence comfortable or unpleasant?

- What was the client expressing non-verbally during the period of silence?

Note down your answers in your diary.

Were you able to distinguish between a comfortable and an uncomfortable silence? If the silence was broken by you, was it because you felt uncomfortable or was it because you honestly felt that the client wanted the silence broken? Some people feel very uncomfortable with silence — but silence, like listening, shows that you respect and care for the other person.

Times when you might have nothing to say

We all know that not all clients can be cured. Some people suffer from diseases for which there is no cure. This can be a shock not only for the client but also for the nurse, who can be left feeling that there is little that can be done or said to help the client cope.

We have all experienced deep feelings of helplessness from time to time. If we have no answers, how can we help the client cope? We have already seen that 'just keeping talking' will not be helpful; we know that we should listen, but sometimes there is no talking to listen to. How do we care about a client in this situation? It is at such times that the nurse's silence might be the most beneficial course of action for the client. Silence can be an active intervention. It is not an abandonment of care; in fact it can be extremely hard work. Consider the following case study.

Mrs Peters had had a long history of intestinal problems, and she had recently been admitted for an exploratory laparotomy. It was established that she had widespread cancer, including liver involvement, and that no curative treatment was possible. After the surgery Mrs Peters asked the doctor to tell her what he had found, making it clear that she wanted to know the truth. The doctor was obviously uncomfortable, being aware that Mrs Peters was only 35 and that she had a young family. He told her the truth, as she had asked, and then left shortly afterwards.

It was clear to the nurse that Mrs Peters needed help, but what could she say? Were there any reassuring words that could be offered? The nurse was aware of her own feelings of helplessness and was almost frozen to the spot on which she stood.

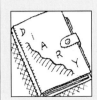

ACTIVITY 6
10 mins
Have you ever been in this sort of situation? What do you think the nurse could have done to be supportive? Share your experiences with a colleague.

Record your thoughts in your diary.

It is quite possible that Mrs Peters just needed someone to be with her. She knew that there were no magic answers, but it would have helped her if she had had real human contact while coming to terms with her situation.

In considering this case study you may well have discovered that it would be difficult not to think along the lines of 'What if this were me in this situation? How would I cope?' It is quite natural to identify with the client in this way, so this may be one of the reasons why some nurses avoid this sort of contact. It tends to remind us all that we are mortal, and this is very painful. Thoughts like this can help us care by putting us in touch with the client. On the other hand, these thoughts can get in the way of genuine caring. No one can know how helpful they might be until they try.

Silence is a risk, because it is one of the hardest forms of communication. However, it *is* communication, and there can be a great deal of non-verbal contact which can communicate very clearly the message: 'You matter, you deserve time and space, I will make no demands of you, I will just be with you'. In Section 2 we suggested that mental health nursing required *being* something rather than simply *doing* something. The case of Mrs Peters is an obvious example of just that.

It must be emphasised that no nurse can offer support to this extent unless he/she feels supported. It is vital that all nurses and managers recognise this need and aim to construct networks of support.

In this Section we have considered some basic skills which might be used in providing psychosocial care. The skills may, at first glance, seem simple but you have probably discovered that this is not so. However, they are the hallmarks of the professional nurse.

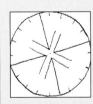

FOCUS
2 hours
Look back at the case studies of Mrs Brown, John Smithson and Mrs Peters.

Do you remember any incidents similar to those experienced by these three people where you believe you were not using your communication skills as well as you might have?

Write a brief account of the incidents in your diary and then outline what you would do differently now, and why.

4. Professional aspects of mental health nursing

This Section is largely concerned with the structures in which mental health nursing takes place and the relationships between the various professional practitioners and other services, including the voluntary sector. Professional and policy issues will also be considered in the light of their effects upon the provision of mental health care.

Community or institutionally-based care?

> Fred Williams' wife, Elsie, had been suffering from a dementing illness for the past three years. He had been caring for her at home with some support but was becoming increasingly exhausted. It was obvious to all that Elsie required residential care but Fred said that he had promised to remain with her 'in sickness and in health' and that is exactly what he intended to do.

Elsie Williams was suffering from a chronic and progressive mental disorder. If Fred had been considering agreeing to place Elsie in residential care there would have been several available options. In the past, Elsie would almost certainly have been accommodated in a continuing care ward in a psychiatric hospital; today, the wisdom of such a measure has been closely examined.

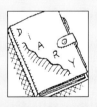

ACTIVITY 1
10-15 mins
What issues do you think should be taken into consideration when contemplating the sort of treatment Elsie should receive? Make some notes in your diary.

There are a number of points of view which need to be taken into account in considering Elsie's case:

• The best interests of Fred and Elsie

• The cost of provision of residential care — it is usually argued that this type of care is poor value for money because large sums are consumed in providing 'hotel services' in outmoded hospitals and relatively little is spent on the provision of actual care and treatment

• The widely held but debatable view that clients like Elsie do not require the skilled intervention of highly-trained professional staff (again, there are cost implications to consider)

- The fact that all too often elderly mentally ill people are accommodated in poor quality environments within hospitals and are often looked after by unqualified staff for long periods. (The care given by these staff may, of course, be adequate or excellent, in which case the issue of appropriateness of accommodation becomes even more pressing — why care for a person in hospital if the skills of hospital-based staff are not indicated?)

Many of the changes in attitudes about the care of mentally ill people have been motivated by national policy, most notably the report of Sir Roy Griffiths, *Agenda for Action*[1], and the government's White Papers, *Working for Patients*[2] and *Caring for People*[3], which preceded the more recent legislation in the NHS and Community Care Act 1990.

Alternatives to continuing care wards in hospitals include nursing and rest homes provided by the NHS, social services and the private sector. In addition, the possibility of providing care and support in the client's own home should not be forgotten[4,5].

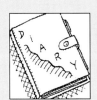

ACTIVITY 2
15-20 mins
Do you think that elderly mentally ill people require the services of qualified nurses? Note down some arguments both for and against.

Discuss this issue with some of your colleagues, and make notes in your diary about any different opinions you meet.

You have probably discovered that many nurses believe that elderly mentally ill people do require the skills of qualified nurses. When asked for justifications, however, nurses are often hard pushed to identify skills other than basic care in relation to physical needs. This sort of care could be provided in a variety of settings and it is easy to suggest, perhaps quite wrongly, that the skills of mental health nurses are not required.

The challenges presented by this area of nursing, however, have led to a resurgence of interest in caring for this client group, and their relatives. It is often the case that relatives like Fred are in need of a great deal of support, both practical and psychological. This support can be provided through groups facilitated by professionals, including mental health nurses. Such nurses are also increasingly trying to maximise the quality of life of elderly people suffering from degenerative mental illness.

Mental or physical care?

Elderly people, perhaps more than any other group, epitomise the need for holistic nursing care. General nurses caring for elderly people often find that their clients are in need of mental health care, and mental health nurses find that their clients are often elderly people who also need general nursing care. In previous Sections you have explored the need to provide care for the 'whole' person. In the light of this, consider the following Activity.

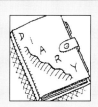

ACTIVITY 3
10-15 mins
What do you think would be the effects on standards of care of creating a specialist group of nurses for care of the elderly?

Make some notes in your diary about the advantages and disadvantages of such a proposal.

The biggest risk associated with the idea of special nurses for elderly people is that they might not receive the same quality of care and treatment as other people who just happen to be younger. (This is an example of ageism.)

On the other hand, it might be argued that, in some cases, elderly people do receive lower standards of care, therefore specialisation could lead to higher commitment and consequent higher standards of care.

It is clear, however, that all nurses should be able to offer a range of basic care to all clients regardless of age and regardless of whether that basic care is primarily psychological or physical.

People who have acute mental disorders

You have probably heard suggestions that seriously mentally ill people are not being properly cared for in hospital. In fact some people argue that they are not being cared for at all![6] As a citizen you may well be concerned and, equally, as a professional you may well have direct experience of the problems, particularly if you have worked in an accident and emergency department. Why does it seem so difficult to arrange for people who are clearly mentally ill to be admitted to a psychiatric hospital?

The following example of the situation of John Brown will help to identify the problems that can arise.

> John Brown's mother became increasingly concerned about her son. He had recently started isolating himself and looked constantly anguished. John himself was surprisingly lucid and described feelings of peculiar detachment as though he were some sort of shadow or spirit. He said that it just felt as though he was asleep and dreaming and would wake up soon.

John was acutely ill and required treatment and care from professional practitioners. What options of care are available?

One option would be to admit him to a psychiatric hospital, but this might not be advised for fear of his becoming institutionalised[7,8]. Another option would be to allow him to receive entirely community-based care, or he could be admitted to a small in-patient unit near his home.

Unfortunately, any delay in deciding on appropriate care for John could cause him to be left with chronic mental health problems for which he might never receive appropriate treatment. He could then pass into a phase where his primary needs are considered as being social — thus casting doubt upon the appropriateness of continuing care from NHS mental health services. In this event his case might be considered to have much in common that of with Elsie, whom we mentioned on page 31.

In cases such as these, the voluntary sector is often able to provide appropriate support to sufferers and their families[9].

ACTIVITY 4
1-2 hours
Find out more about the range of voluntary and statutory mental health-care provision in your area. Try to identify the roles of the National Schizophrenia Fellowship, Mind, the Alzheimer's Disease Society and other voluntary organisations — your local hospital and library services should help you. Try to establish the range of statutory services in your area; how might they address the needs of Fred Williams or Mrs Brown?

Add the information you collect to your community profile.

Institutionalisation is a serious side-effect of institutional care, although it is not the only reason why care is increasingly being offered in the community. Most professionals agree that there is much to be done in improving the quality of community care. But if improvements take place it might well be that impressions of 'abandonment in the community' and 'relegation to an institution' will both disappear in favour of real care and concern for mentally ill people.

Admission and treatment: The role of the Mental Health Act 1983

It is a commonly held but largely mistaken belief that the Mental Health Act 1983 is intended to facilitate treatment and hospitalisation where clients refuse such measures. It could be argued, however, that the Act is designed to ensure that the rights of mentally ill people are protected, as it makes clear provision for informal admission to hospital for treatment (Section 131). (Previous legislation had required patients to be certified in order to gain admission and treatment.) The Act also makes it clear that informal patients have the same status as other hospital patients: they can consent to or refuse treatment and they can leave hospital if they wish.

The nature of mental illness, particularly serious illness, is such that some patients who might most benefit from hospital admission and treatment are the least likely to seek admission. In brief it might be suggested that some patients, by virtue of their illness, lack the necessary insight to seek care and treatment. It would be an irony if ill people could not gain treatment because they were ill! The Mental Health Act aims to address this irony by providing facility for:

• Admission for assessment (Section 2)
• Admission for treatment (Section 3)
• Detention of an informal patient (Section 5.2 — doctor's holding power; Section 5.4 — nurse's holding power)
• Treatment where the patient is unable to consent (Part 4).

The Act also protects the rights of detained patients by providing access to mental health review tribunals which make an independent review of alleged unjustified detention in hospital. Furthermore, detained patients are visited by members of the Mental Health Act Commission who review the operation of the Act and ensure that the rights of the patients are respected.

Part 3 of the Mental Health Act is concerned with the treatment and care of patients who are also subject to criminal proceedings.

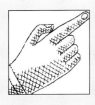

ACTIVITY 5
2 hours
The above summary of the Mental Health Act 1983 is a brief overview. Take this opportunity to read about the Act in more detail. An excellent account of the Mental Health Acts of the United Kingdom and Eire is provided by Killen[10].

Having explored some of the practical and policy issues relating to providing care for the mentally ill, we end the module by considering some of the professional issues. What is the significance of what we have said in this module for nursing as a profession, and for general nurses in particular?

General nursing and mental health nursing: the case for mutual understanding

The case of Gladys Miles, which was discussed in Section 2, provides a good example of the different orientations of general and mental health nurses, so we repeat it here.

> Gladys Miles, a 58-year-old single woman, was referred for radical mastectomy following positive diagnosis of carcinoma. She believed strongly that the consequent disfigurement would be so severe that the treatment would be best avoided. A nurse was asked to talk with Gladys to help her make an informed choice.

Gladys' case provides a good example of the need for teamwork in the provision of health care. A doctor diagnosed Gladys' condition and provided a plan of treatment, but it was most likely that nurses (general and mental health) would have been the recipients of most of her questions. A specialist nurse, general nurses, physiotherapists and a surgical appliance specialist would all have been involved in her care and all these people would have needed to work closely together in order to provide Gladys with optimal care and treatment.

Gladys' case also highlights some interesting legal and ethical issues. It is Gladys' right to refuse treatment, even if it is life-saving. The fact that she has refused should not be taken as evidence of mental illness. She may or may not be ill. It is, of course, the duty of the nurse to enable Gladys to make informed choices, but it is an abrogation of duty to attempt to compel Gladys to accept treatment against her better judgement. Caring about Gladys may well lead the nurse to accept her decision even though the nurse might regard it as foolish.

Acceptance of a person and the decisions he/she makes is a familiar concept in mental health nursing. Some general nurses would regard Gladys and her refusal of treatment as a problem to be dealt with by mental health nurses. Assuming that Gladys is not mentally ill, nothing could be further from the truth.

The major difference between the two groups of nurses is that mental health nurses are more likely to try to understand Gladys' decision, whereas it might be incomprehensible to some general nurses, who will be more concerned with attempting to change it. This is not intended to be a criticism; it is a reflection of the differences in training received by nurses in different specialties.

There have been few examples of general and mental health nurses working together in the past, although there are examples of notable developments in such areas as liaison nursing. This may be because the two groups see their roles differently, or it might just be a reflection of their different training. There has been an attempt to address some of these problems in Project 2000[11]. At present, the client is all too often the loser; Gladys might not have been mentally ill at all, but there is little doubt that she could have benefited from mental health nursing skills if they were available.

Does Project 2000 help to bridge the gap between the two groups?

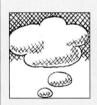

ACTIVITY 6
30 mins
Look at the recommendations in Professional Paper 9, 'The Final Proposals', of Project 2000[12].

- **Do you think that this style of training helps nurses to care for the 'whole person'?**

- **Do you think that it will better enable nurses to understand each other's roles?**

You have probably discovered from your reading that Project 2000 includes a recommendation that all nurses should undertake an initial period of training together. It is likely that this period of shared training will assist all nurses to become skilled in a range of interventions which will help clients such as Gladys.

What is the role of the mental health nurse?

It might be argued that, perhaps 50 years ago, the respective roles of general and mental health nurses were very different. In the case of the latter, they were still regarded as 'lunatic attendants'. After the 1940s, however, the two roles appear to have become increasingly similar, particularly as those previously identified as 'insane', for instance, gradually came to be understood as ill and in need of treatment[13,14].

In more recent times, however, it would seem that the mental health nurse is losing a nursing identity in favour of that of a practitioner with a therapeutic orientation. Some people argue that mental health nurses have more in common with colleagues practising in mental health (for example, social workers, psychologists and occupational therapists) than nurses practising in other branches of nursing.

So what do mental health nurses do? The following case studies may help you to understand the role of the mental health nurse.

James Smith complained of an increasing lack of concentration. He felt lifeless and purposeless despite having developed a successful career as a draughtsman. He denied that there were any problems in his life; indeed, he claimed that many would envy his successful social situation. However, he was very aware that something was amiss but did not know where to start in trying to sort out the problem.

Although Robert Briggs did not have a particularly eventful sex life, he was convinced that he was HIV positive and demanded an AIDS test. It was revealed that Robert had had a brief homosexual relationship in late adolescence but that there had been no penetrative intercourse. By now he had a steady heterosexual relationship but was evading his girlfriend's hints about marriage because of his belief that he had AIDS.

Clients such as James Smith and Robert Briggs are unlikely to require in-patient treatment, but they may benefit from individual counselling within the framework of an effective nurse–client relationship. It is possible that they might be referred directly to a nurse, as is increasingly happening, partly in recognition of the wide range of skilled intervention which many mental health nurses are able to offer.

There are now many examples of autonomous practice in mental health nursing; referrals are often made to a team of practitioners and the team member most able to help the particular client takes responsibility for the case. This approach does not mean that the client is denied access to other team members (for example, if James were found to be suffering from serious depressive illness, it would be clear that he would require medical help and his case would be referred on).

It is clear from the discussion above that the role of the mental health nurse has changed considerably in recent times. It is often suggested that there are three main aspects to the mental health nurse's role:

1. *Custodial*, where the emphasis is upon accommodating the mentally ill person in safety, either for the benefit of the client or in the interests of other members of society.

2. *Procedural*, including largely the delivery of basic nursing care (for example, the giving of injections).

3. *Therapeutic*, where the nurse is directly involved in the treatment of a mentally ill person. This may be through the management of a therapeutic relationship, or it might include the use of specific therapeutic techniques, such as counselling and psychotherapy. It should

be emphasised that the nurse is not necessarily a counsellor, though counselling approaches might be within the context of the nurse-client relationship. The development of this role is clearly explained by Reynolds and Cormack[15].

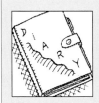

ACTIVITY 7
1 hour
Discuss the above analysis of the mental health nurse's role with an experienced mental health nurse, noting in particular the changing emphasis of these three aspects over the past 10 years.

You should not assume that this role analysis differentiates mental health and general nursing. Custodial care was common in all branches of nursing in the past. Consider, for example, the role of the nurse in the care of chronically disabled clients and those suffering from infectious disease before the advent of antibiotic drugs.

Similarly, there is evidence to suggest that, increasingly, the general nurse is developing a therapeutic orientation in terms of the psychosocial and other aspects of her role. The evolving role of the general nurse who is also employed as a specialist is of particular relevance here — the stoma nurse, for example.

Responsibilities in mental health nursing

Mental health nursing often leads the nurse to become involved with clients' families. Sometimes this highlights considerable responsibilities. Consider the following case study.

Tony Drummond asked for help at an alcohol advice centre. He was quite clear that although he was not an alcoholic he tended to drink heavily when under stress and then become violent towards his wife and children. He was seriously worried that his family was at risk.

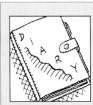

ACTIVITY 8
30 mins
Imagine that Tony had mentioned his problems to a nurse.

• What should a nurse do when confronted by such an alarming problem?

• If Tony's wife and family were at risk and he had the courage to seek help, what form should this take?

Make some notes in your diary.

Tony said that he was not an alcoholic, yet there is a tendency to regard people such as him as though they were because they continue to drink when, by their own admission, there is a clear need to stop. In this case it is likely that Tony was reluctant to call himself an alcoholic partly because he feared rejection by friends, family and professionals

PART 1:4

and partly because he did not see himself as fitting into the stereotype of a 'drunken down and out'. However, Tony had already crossed the first hurdle in admitting that he had a problem.

Tony could well have benefited from specialist help available through either the health service or the voluntary sector. In the initial stages it would be crucial to ensure that Tony was not judged and that the trust that he had invested was respected. In this situation the nurse is probably unable to offer any long-term solutions to problems like Tony's and further help should be sought from other health professionals.

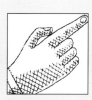

ACTIVITY 9
1-2 hours
What are the prevalent attitudes in your area of work towards people with alcohol problems? Does the stereotype prevail or are people willing to admit that this is a problem that can affect anyone?

Are there any special policies in your health district regarding the management of staff with alcohol problems? Take advantage of this opportunity to learn more about the work of Alcoholics Anonymous and Al-Anon in your own area.

Gather information from as many local sources as you can to help you carry out this Activity, and record your findings in your community profile.

People who have alcohol-or drug-related problems nearly always require the combined expertise of professional staff from both general and mental health services as well as help from voluntary organisations. You will probably have discovered this situation when investigating your own area.

Summary

This Section has been concerned with the management and organisation of mental health services. You should now be aware of some of the arguments for and against community care and the effects of policy change in this area from the client's point of view. The changing role of the mental health nurse has also been considered, particularly as it affects other nurses. Throughout this Section there has been a recurrent theme of the benefits of teamwork, including involvement of the voluntary sector. Perhaps the most important message is that all nurses need basic mental health knowledge and skills in order to ensure that the care of all clients is properly managed.

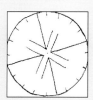

FOCUS
2 hours
Look back at the three clients whose psychosocial care you considered in Activity 1 of Section 1.

As a result of working through this module, write in your diary any changes in these clients' planned psychosocial care which you would now consider to be appropriate, and explain your reasons.

Alternatively, you may prefer to consider three different clients when carrying out this Focus Activity.

1. Difficulties, disabilities and disadvantages

Introduction

In Part II of this module we will be discussing issues and ideas associated with learning disability. We begin by introducing some of the main ideas which influence contemporary thinking about services for people with learning disabilities. We then explore the current concepts in the area and look at the implications of terminology and definitions associated with the provision of services, and at the relationship between impairment, disability and handicap.

The importance of language

As human beings we have a unique capacity to make sense of our experience by creating meaning. This is a consequence of our highly sophisticated nervous system and our ability to use language. Words, phrases and sentences, the building blocks of language, enable us to convert our private thoughts into communication with others. They also provide the means by which we learn to describe and understand ourselves, other people and the world in which we live. We not only exchange information but we also communicate attitudes, values and beliefs.

We use language to explain how we are feeling and to express opinions on what we like and don't like. What, then, should we make of the following report?

> At a conference on the subject of 'learning disabilities' a person rose to give his talk. Printed on his T-shirt were the words 'LABELS ARE FOR JARS — NOT PEOPLE'. The person speaking explained that he received services for people who have a mental handicap but pointed out that there is nothing *mental* about him. He reminded the audience that he is only *handicapped* because society has restricted his opportunities and choices. The speaker mentioned the difficulties he experiences in learning new things and applying new knowledge. For this reason he suggested that it would be more appropriate for people to describe him as 'a person with a learning difficulty'.

This story not only illustrates the importance of language but also highlights several issues which are central to this part of the module:

• There are different opinions on whether 'learning difficulty', 'learning disability' or 'mental handicap' is the best way of describing the nature of problems experienced by people who require special services because of their inability to learn as fast or as well as other people

• Particular words, such as 'mental', can have unintended associations which affect how a term is understood

- Unlike an inanimate object, such as a 'jar', a person who is described by means of a particular term (or label) can have a view on the language which is used

- Service-users can (and do) discuss aspects of the services which they are receiving and as 'consumers' are able to provide perspectives which are different from those of professionals.

The point that the speaker was making — that the phrase 'learning difficulty' is more acceptable to him than 'mental handicap' — suggests that as professionals we need to be willing to review and amend the terms which we use.

Our language is shaped by many social and cultural factors. However, as nurses it is important that we should be aware if words and phrases which we use are offensive to particular people.

One of the main problems with the term 'mental handicap' has been the tendency for confusion in the media between 'mental handicap' and 'mental illness'.

Convincing arguments have been put forward that either 'learning difficulty' or 'learning disability' should replace the term 'mental handicap'. 'Learning difficulty' is the term most commonly used by service users, although even those using it often recognise it as imperfect. This is because it presents the issue as simply a problem of slow learning. This, in turn, implies that a 'good dose of education' is the 'cure'. It also highlights the fact that this particular group of people differs from others only in the extent to which they face problems in coping with life in a highly technical society. We all find learning difficult in certain circumstances.

ACTIVITY 1
5 minutes
Think about what you would need to learn to be able to carry out the following three tasks and estimate how long it would take you to complete each one:

- Write down the rules for playing a game of hockey

- Translate this sentence into Albanian

- Memorise and recall accurately the sequence of playing cards in a shuffled pack.

Clearly, the length of time that it would take you to complete the first two tasks will depend on your existing knowledge. If you know the rules of hockey you will be able to complete the first task fairly quickly. Similarly, if you can already translate English into Albanian the second task will be relatively easy. If you don't already know the rules of hockey and can't translate English into Albanian you will still be able to complete the tasks if you are able to acquire the relevant knowledge. For most people, learning the rules of hockey will be easier than learning to translate English into Albanian.

Of course, to complete the first of these Activities you will need to have mastered the complex skill of writing and to complete the second you will need to understand two languages. In the case of the third task you don't have to be able to read and write or understand language but will need to be able to memorise and recall accurately a sequence of 52 images.

When you carried out the Activity you probably considered:
1. What you already knew and how it would make these tasks easy or difficult.
2. The effort it would take for you to acquire the necessary pre-requisite knowledge.
3. The extent to which your ability to memorise and recall could cope with the demands of the tasks (particularly the third).

If your estimate of the time that it would take you to complete these three tasks is longer than that of others, does it mean you have a learning difficulty? No. All three of the tasks would generally be viewed as very difficult. Consequently, no matter how long you think you will take to do them, these activities would not be appropriate as a means of assessing whether or not you have a learning difficulty.

In fact, it is more likely that people who are able to complete these tasks faster than others would be considered to be 'clever', 'talented', 'gifted' or 'a genius'. The world record for memorising and recalling the sequence of playing cards in a shuffled pack is less than two minutes. Feel free to try and beat this time if you wish!

The capacity to learn is a highly valued personal characteristic in contemporary society. Generally, people like to be told that they are 'clever', 'talented', 'gifted', 'bright' or 'intelligent'. These are characteristics which people would tend to rate positively.

Similarly, there are very many words and phrases in common usage which are used negatively to describe people who have difficulty learning. Most people have experience of being called 'stupid', 'dull', 'dim', 'slow' or 'thick' at some time in their lives. Even worse, terms such as 'idiot', 'imbecile' and 'moron', which are now commonly used terms of abuse, were introduced into our language at different times to describe people with varying degrees of learning difficulties.

Terms which preceded 'mental handicap', but which have been rejected as inappropriate because of negative associations, include 'mental subnormality', 'mental retardation' and 'mental deficiency'. It should come as no surprise, therefore, that 'you're just an LD' as a derogatory comment has already been heard in a playground.

Learning disability: an explanation

Everyone will experience difficulty in learning unless he or she already has the necessary knowledge for the task in hand. Generally, however, for someone to be said to have a learning difficulty there must be an identified problem in the individual's capacity to process information.

The nature and extent of 'information processing' problems which people can experience may vary considerably[1]. An individual can have a very specific learning difficulty such as dyslexia, characterised by difficulty in processing written information, though the capacity to learn via auditory channels remains unaffected. Alternatively, a learning difficulty may be so widespread and complete that throughout the person's lifetime he or she is unable to acquire knowledge to a level which would be regarded as normal for a young child.

When an individual's learning difficulty is sufficiently general and sufficiently severe to interfere with his or her ability to cope with ordinary daily activities, it is normally referred to as a *learning disability*. In this module you will explore some of the issues which arise in providing services for this group of people and their families. It is worth noting that the term *mental handicap*, which is still in use, can be used interchangeably with the term learning disability.

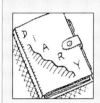

ACTIVITY 2
10 minutes
How has your current understanding of the problems experienced by people with learning disabilities and their families developed?

• Make a list in your diary of the experiences which you consider to have shaped your thinking.

You may be close to someone with a learning disability, perhaps in your own family or group of friends. Or you may be friendly with someone who has a child with a learning disability. You may have worked with people with learning disabilities who have health problems, and will probably have encountered items in the media which discuss this area from a medical or social perspective.

All these experiences will have contributed to your current understanding of problems faced by people with learning disabilities. This knowledge and understanding will continue to develop and be influenced by your experiences and encounters with people with learning disability.

It may be particularly useful to think about the similarities and differences between having a learning disability and another kind of disability.

In developing a framework of definitions for use by the World Health Organisation, Wood[2] clarified differences in the meanings of the terms 'impairment', 'disability' and 'handicap':

• *Impairment* is used to describe a loss or limitation in an individual's bodily part or mechanism

• *Disability* describes the restrictions on the individual's functional ability which arise as a consequence of impairment

• *Handicap* refers to the social disadvantage which accrues as a result of an individual's impairment or disability.

The impairment of an individual's developing nervous system, which may be the result of damage before, during or after birth, will inhibit the development of normal learning abilities and result in a disability. A person with a learning disability is handicapped by the extent to which his or her opportunities to fulfil roles within society (commensurate with age, sex and social and cultural factors) are restricted.

The classification system adopted by the World Health Organisation is not in general use — the terms, impairment, disability and handicap are still used interchangeably — but it has been the focus of considerable debate. In particular, objections have been raised to the idea that disability is solely something to do with an individual's functioning rather than society's response to the problems associated with an impairment. As an alternative, Oliver[3] defines disability as 'socially imposed restriction' and Finkelstein and French[4] have suggested that it is useful to consider disability as the loss or limitation of opportunities that prevents people who have impairments from taking part in the normal life of the community on an equal level with others owing to physical and social barriers.

Discussions about definitions of disability are not simply about terminology. In developing services for people with impairments, much will depend on where the emphasis is placed. Is it on improving an individual's functional ability or on altering physical and social environments to enable participation in everyday activities?

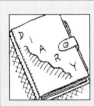

ACTIVITY 3
20 minutes
Imagine that you have an impairment which means that you are unable to walk.

• Note down in your diary the actions which others would need to take to enable you to retain your current lifestyle.

You may have identified the need for help in ensuring your house and local neighbourhood are made barrier free; or the assistance you would require to get access to equipment which would allow you to retain as much independence as possible. You may also have listed the help you would need to obtain a source of income which would allow you to continue with your current spending pattern, or to maintain your range of leisure activities.

The active participation of a wide range of people (including town planners, housing providers, product designers and employers) is required if people with disabilities are to achieve ordinary lifestyles. At present, however, the particular requirements of people with disabilities are not usually taken into account when decisions are taken.

Advocacy

In recent times there has been a growing disabled people's rights movement. Campaigners with disabilities have sought to change the idea that they are deserving of charity towards the view that everyone in society should have the right to participate in, and contribute to, their local communities. This approach emphasises the development of equal opportunities policies and practices and the ending of discrimination, which is so commonly experienced by people with disabilities.

People with learning disabilities have been less active in campaigning for 'rights' than, for instance, people with visual or physical disabilities. However, the social disadvantage and discrimination experienced by people with an impaired ability to learn are considerable handicaps. It is within this context that the development of citizen advocacy schemes and the encouragement of self-advocacy are seen as essential components of service provision for adults with learning disabilities[5].

ACTIVITY 4
30 minutes
Spend up to 15 minutes on each of the following:

• Self-advocacy aims to encourage people to speak up for themselves, make choices and take decisions. It is something which most of us take for granted. What everyday choices or decisions have you made during the past 24 hours (for example when to go to bed or what to have for breakfast)? Make a list of about 10.

• Citizen advocacy schemes aim to match each service-user with a volunteer who will act as his or her advocate. The advocate is an ordinary citizen rather than a professional or a relative of the service-user. Can you think of an occasion when a fellow citizen spoke up on your behalf?

• Make notes in your diary.

You were probably able to list many everyday decisions — every time you buy something (or decide not to buy), go somewhere (or decide not to go) or do something (or decide not to do it), you are exercising choice. It is also possible that you took a major decision over the past 24 hours which will affect many aspects of your life — deciding to look for a new house, for example, or apply for a new job.

People with learning disabilities are often in a situation where other people take decisions on their behalf. This is not necessarily because the person is unable to have an opinion; it is often more to do with making life easier for the carers. However, making choices and taking decisions is an important part of life, and provides opportunities for learning. It is thus important that every effort is made to enable people with learning disabilities to exercise control over their everyday activities.

You may have found it more difficult to think of a situation in which a fellow citizen spoke up on your behalf, though it is likely you will consult friends and colleagues before you take a decision which will entail change in your life. In our society, it is generally expected that adults will be able to find out about their rights and responsibilities and speak up for themselves. However, if you are a member of a campaigning group, a trade union or political party there will be formal arrangements for selecting representatives who have authority to speak on your behalf. Nursing as a profession also has arrangements whereby certain individuals are given authority to represent the views of all nurses.

Many decisions are taken on behalf of people with learning disabilities by professional carers — who consider themselves to be appropriately placed to know what is in the individual's best interest. However, professionals also have to act on behalf of their employers, and there is always the possibility of conflicting interests between the authority and the service-user. Citizen advocacy schemes seek to ensure that people with learning disabilities have access to someone who can provide unbiased representation if required.

Countering disadvantage

The ways in which people with disabilities are viewed have changed. Commenting on the way in which social welfare policies have altered during the course of the 20th century, Alaszewski points to the move from people with learning disabilities being seen as 'villains' to their being characterised as 'victims of past attitudes and inappropriate services'[6]. How people with learning disabilities are represented in the media is becoming more varied. However, there is still a tendency for simplification of complex issues and the construction of stereotypes which minimise individual differences. One study of articles from a newspaper found evidence to support the view that people with learning disabilities tend to be portrayed as 'eternal children' or as 'sick people'[7].

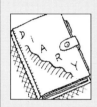

ACTIVITY 5
10 minutes
It is not only people with learning disabilities who are portrayed in a stereotyped way. Consider how nurses are represented in the media and note in your diary some of the common stereotypes which appear.

Our understanding of the world is developed through our own experience, modified by insights gained from a wide variety of sources[8]. Representations that are well-established and continuously reinforced however, can be very difficult to challenge.

The negative images often associated with having a learning disability would suggest that being slower to learn than other people necessarily means that one's life will be 'all doom and gloom'. The reality is that people with learning disabilities can lead interesting and fulfilling lives. Families, friends and professional carers often find that someone with a learning disability is able to provide refreshingly uninhibited responses; sometimes an individual with a learning disability will say what other people would like to say but don't because they have learned that this is 'not the done thing'.

Even when the learning disability is so pervasive that the person is unable to develop language, and remains totally dependent on others for personal care and assistance, it is still possible that he or she will be able to contribute socially by providing inspiration for others.

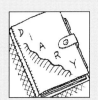

ACTIVITY 6
20 minutes
How does your role as a nurse affect the way in which you think about people with learning disabilities and their families? Note in your diary your responses to the following questions:

- In what ways has being a nurse influenced how you feel about working with someone who has very limited ability to communicate and requires help with all aspects of self-care?

- In what ways has being a nurse influenced how you feel about a mother who has 24-hour responsibility for caring for someone with these problems?

Your role as a nurse will affect how you relate to people who are dependent on others for personal care and who require assistance to carry out even the most basic self-care tasks. It is intrinsic to the profession of nursing and thus reflected in the code of professional conduct that people are treated in a manner which upholds their dignity and personal worth.

In your response to this Activity you may have felt that your role as a nurse enabled you to empathise with family members who are caring for a highly dependent person at home.

It is also likely that you will have been socialised into a working environment based on clear differentiation between health and social care issues. In addition, you may have had experience of working within services which are geared towards 'diagnosis and treatment'. Though people with learning disabilities can experience the same medical problems as other people, and in some instances are more likely to experience particular health problems, their disability is not an illness.

Some of the issues surrounding the creation of relevant and effective health services for people with learning disabilities and their families, and the role of nurses in helping to achieve high-quality local services for people with continuing and complex problems, are addressed more fully in Section 4.

Normalisation

For the reasons cited above the notion of 'normalisation' is often cited as a basis for designing services which can counter the negative images and ideas associated with learning disabilities[9]. Normalisation (which is also referred to as social role valorisation because the intention is 'to create a positive imbalance' or 'to valorise' opportunities for the adoption of valued roles within society) has various shades of meaning with different emphases apparent among its proponents. However, its essential elements are the promotion of social integration and the provision of services which encourage and assist people with learning disabilities to adopt 'ordinary' (or 'normal') lifestyles.

Brechin and Swain[10] comment:

'Some inherent problems remain in a concept premised on the

desirability of normality, in whatever sense it is interpreted. If it is used, however, to highlight commonly experienced deprivations and restrictions, and stimulate a move away from those towards a range of service provisions and life-styles which would normally be seen as more adequate, more acceptable, and even more desirable — which would, in short, be valued by most of society — then normalisation must offer some hope of a breakthrough[9].

ACTIVITY 7
30 minutes
Think of three people who you know quite well (friends or relatives) and write down similarities and differences in their lifestyles under each of the following three headings. We have suggested some factors which could be used for this Activity but you should feel free to include any others.

• Where he or she lives
You may wish to consider: the type of accommodation; where it is located; whether anyone else lives in the same house; size (are there more rooms than people?); decor and furnishings.

• Work and leisure activities
You may wish to consider: whether employed, self-employed or unemployed and status of type of work; the amount of time which the person devotes to work and other activities; whether the person goes out regularly; leisure activities; attitude to holiday arrangements.

• Relationships
You may wish to consider: whether or not the person has chosen to live with a partner; views on marriage; the extent to which contact is maintained with family members; the extent to which he or she socialises with people from work; and the importance which he or she places on 'independence'.

When you have completed your analysis comment on the extent to which each person would consider the others to have a 'normal lifestyle'. Include your findings and your comments in your community profile.

You may have discovered during this Activity that trying to describe a normal or ordinary lifestyle may give rise to many problems. Even though a common cultural and social framework might be discerned, everyone has his/her own idiosyncratic views and personal preferences.

People with learning disabilities generally have to depend on the help and assistance of others if they are to exercise choice in important aspects of everyday life. Support is required to determine where to live, what sort of employment and leisure activities to undertake and to establish a network of contacts and supportive relationships. This means that others — whether they be family members or professional carers — are in a position to exert much more influence over the lifestyles of people with learning disabilities than would be the case for other citizens.

It is within this context that advocacy and normalisation are considered to be important ideas assisting carers to create the sorts of services which can help to promote integration[11]. However, for full social integration to be achieved many individuals, groups and organisations who are not directly involved in working with people with learning disabilities need to take steps to ensure their inclusion in everyday activities. In discussing how the concept of inclusion can be used to influence people's attitude towards fellow citizens with learning disabilities, Jupp[12] outlines a fruitful direction for the future when he comments:

•We have unwittingly relegated some people to a second-class human league by continually concentrating on "doing things to them" rather than "enabling and empowering them" to live the lifestyle of their choice. Somehow, we have become rather adept at mystifying the additional needs of certain children and adults. These, we say, are people who need specialist help, specialist staff, special places; but these "special" places simply turn out to be places which are in fact separate, which segregate them from everyone else. Those people whom we call "special" are the ones we earmark for a life apart•.

Changing attitudes to disability

Disabled people have lived in all societies and through all historical ages. Taking a broad view of events, Finkelstein[13] has identified three main phases in the development of attitudes towards people with disabilities:

1. In mainly rural societies, before the industrial age, people had less need to be mobile. There was no formal education system and no organised medicine. The social system was fairly stable, so disabled people would have remained within their community. Tasks such as cooking, making clothes and helping to care for children could fall well within the capacities of most disabled people.

2. As agricultural machinery became more complex and goods needed to be moved about, the position of disabled people became more tenuous. It could be dangerous, or too difficult, for a disabled person to perform such tasks. The industrial revolution continued this development and mass production techniques meant that machinery had to be designed for the average person. People were now living mainly in towns and had to travel to work. Problems of sanitation and disease created disabilities and so, too, did new industries like coal mining: accidents and respiratory problems were common. Disabled people could not contribute to economic activity and their only means of income was charity; institutions for their care and support began to grow.

3. Disabled people have begun to organise themselves and are asserting their rights. More material and practical help is available and disabled people are increasingly involved in service planning. Disabled people who have been segregated from the rest of society are now being integrated.

In this Section we have looked at the terminology and definitions associated wtih impairment, disability and handicap and have considered Finkelstein's analysis of how economic and social changes over a long period of time have affected how people with disabilities are treated. The following Focus Activity asks you to think about social and economic changes both in your life to date and in the future.

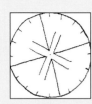

FOCUS
2 hours
Exercise 1 (15 minutes)
Finkelstein's analysis considers how economic and social changes over a long period of time have affected how people with disabilities are treated.

What do you consider are the main social and economic changes which have occurred in your lifetime?

Write down a list of changes and comment on the likely effects that each will have had on the provision of services for people with disabilities.

Exercise 2 (1 hour 45 minutes)
Once you have completed the first exercise think about economic and social changes which are likely to take place in the future and the possible effects of further development of the third phase which Finkelstein has identified.

Imagine that you are living in the year 2050 and are describing the services which a person with a particular disability is receiving.

Write an essay of 500 words from this perspective (remembering to make clear what the nature of the disability is that you are discussing).

2. Children and families

In this Section we explore some of the issues which arise in relation to the provision of services for children with learning disabilities living at home. The initial impact of discovering that a child has a learning disability is considered, and families' experiences of home life and schooling are examined.

Part of the family

Family life is an experience common to most of us. The vast majority of children, including those with learning disabilities, are cared for within the family until they leave school and set up homes of their own. Everyone starts life being totally dependent on others for survival, though for a child with a learning disability the rate at which his or her capacity for independent action develops will be slower than would be expected under normal circumstances. How much slower will depend on many factors - including, crucially, the severity of the impairment. An additional factor, however, which will influence the child's development, is the way in which the family functions.

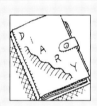

ACTIVITY 1
5 minutes
What images come into your mind when you think of the word 'family'?

Concentrate on this for a moment then write down in your diary all the words that come into your mind.

Representations of an 'ideal' family life tend to be a very powerful influence. The media bombard us daily with images of a 'cereal package' existence and every political party claims to be the one to uphold 'traditional family values'. Some see the family as the basic building block of society. A family can be a symbol of security, the home a place in which tensions can be relieved. Families can also be seen to be the principal means of fulfilling the physical, emotional and social needs of their members.

The family performs an important function in teaching children how to become members of society. Worsley[1] illustrates how the family mediates between the individual and society: the influences of society on an individual are 'filtered' through the family. Similarly, individual members' concerns and aspirations can be channelled into society via the family.

The popular image of the family group is of a mother, father and two children. In reality, of course, families are diverse. Children are now cared for by one or two partners who may or may not be married; other relatives may share the home; one or both parents may be employed or unemployed; brothers and sisters may live together or in different homes. Whatever the family is, it is certainly not a fixed or static concept.

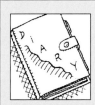

ACTIVITY 2
15 minutes
Think about your own family.

• Try to remember an event in your family that caused a certain amount of stress or tension. Consider which people were principally affected by this event and how other members of the family reacted.

• Write a short account (around 300 words) in your diary.

Within each family, members will have different roles. Are you a parent or grandparent? Whether you are or not, you are someone's son or daughter. You may be someone's brother or sister, uncle or aunt. You may also have a less formal role in your family (for example 'the joker' or 'the thoughtful one'). These roles will change over the years.

Families have to adapt to inevitable and essential changes, such as moves of house, changes in jobs, and alterations in routines. Rather than just being a collection of individuals, a family can be considered as a dynamic system. Anything which happens to one member of a family will also have repercussions for other members.

It is worth making the point that children with learning disabilities are born into *ordinary* families. Although the effects on family members will vary depending on individual circumstances, it is inevitable that each member will be affected by the discovery that a child is slow to learn in some academic and social pursuits. The point when problems are detected will vary. Sometimes parents are aware before the child's birth that he or she will have a learning disability; in other cases it is shortly after birth. Some parents receive confirmation that their child has difficulties only after a period of months or years and, in some instances, the child's normal developmental progress will be halted by accident or illness.

In view of the range of possible causes of a child's impaired ability to learn, and because of the difficulty in ascertaining the nature and extent of individual problems, it is difficult to record accurately the number of children who have a learning disability. It is generally agreed that between 2 and 3% of the population have learning difficulties which are of sufficient extent to affect their ability to cope with aspects of everyday life. However, it is a relatively small proportion of this group of people who have the severest learning disabilities[2].

In many cases the cause of a child's impaired ability to learn is not known. However, if it is associated with a chromosomal abnormality such as Down syndrome, this will be readily identified. Tests carried out during pregnancy can, with various degrees of accuracy, show the presence of additional genetic material in the cells of the unborn child, which is indicative of this condition. Moreover, the characteristic appearance of a child with Down syndrome will normally be apparent at the time of birth and can be confirmed by tests. Down syndrome is the most commonly occurring known chromosomal abnormality causing learning disability, though there are other conditions which have similar aetiology.

Several inherited genetic abnormalities and metabolic disorders are known to cause impaired ability to learn and during pregnancy a number of factors are known to have the potential to affect adversely the central nervous system of the unborn child. These include: the effects of alcohol or drug misuse; poor nutrition; and infections such as rubella.

Furthermore, damage can occur during birth — for instance if the child is starved of oxygen through prolonged occlusion of the umbilical cord — and, in the early years of life, infection or accident can also result in the child's having a learning disability.

The social environment in which a child is brought up will play a part in determining how well adaption can be made to the demands of everyday life. Within this context neglect or ill-treatment can result in delayed development of the child's intellectual functioning. Equally, an environment which provides stimulation, encouragement, support and love will enable the child to develop at a rate which is commensurate with his or her potential.

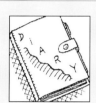

ACTIVITY 3
40 minutes
There are often complex ethical issues associated with the birth of a child with a learning disability. Consider the following scenarios, which are all actual incidents which occurred during the 1980s.

1. The father of a baby with Down syndrome was charged with her murder. In a study of attitudes Sinson[3] asked members of the public what they thought should be the outcome of the trial. Twenty-six per cent of mothers felt that even if Mr Brown were found guilty he should not be punished as severely as if he had murdered a 'normal' child.

2. A girl born with Down syndrome also had an intestinal obstruction. Doctors proposed an operation to save the girl's life but her parents refused to give consent. The child was made a ward of court with the local authority and consent was given to the operation taking place.

3. A paediatrician withheld treatment from a newly born boy with Down syndrome after his parents had appeared to reject the child. The doctor was charged with attempted murder but was acquitted by the jury, who appeared to accept that the child had a poor chance of survival.

• What ethical dilemmas are apparent within each of these scenarios?

• In your opinion, what would you say are the 'rights and wrongs' in each situation?

Note your responses in your diary.

Learning to cope

Regardless of how good or bad the experience of bringing up a child with a learning disability is likely to be, the initial reaction of parents to the news that their child has a condition associated with impaired learning is quite possibly going to be characterised by disappointment and dejection. Cunningham and Davies[4] suggest that many parents have feelings of grief similar to those felt when a close relative dies. This bereavement is brought on by the symbolic 'loss' of the expected 'normal' child — a child who would be expected to be perfect in every way. They describe this process in their model of 'psychic crisis' which provides a framework to help explain emotional responses. Cunningham and Davies identify the following phases:

- *Shock phase*: Emotional disorganisation, confusion, paralysis of actions, disbelief and irrationality. (This can last from two minutes to seven days)

- *Reaction phase*: Expression of sorrow, grief, disappointment, anxiety, aggression, denial, guilt, failure, defence mechanisms

- *Adaption phase*: Realistic appraisal — parents ask: 'What can be done?' This is a signal of readiness to proceed with: 'How can we help?'

- *Orientation phase*: Parents begin to organise, seek help and information, plan for the future.

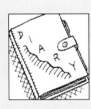

ACTIVITY 4
30 minutes
Think about the last time you received news which upset you.

- Did someone tell you the news or did you find out in some other way? If you were told, what did the person do or say to try to make it easier for you to take the news?

- Were your emotional responses in any way similar to the phases described above by Cunningham and Davies?

Write down your responses in your diary.

One person responded to this Activity by recalling his wife telling him of his mother's death. He remembers his wife being very upset herself, which appeared to help because someone was sharing in his grief. He was told in a quiet area of his workplace, which made him comfortable about expressing his initial shock. His young daughter was also present and he believed that this was important as he wanted his family around him. His colleagues were told soon afterwards and they immediately assured him that they could cope if he was away for any length of time.

There can be no ideal way of informing parents that their child has a learning disability. However, if there is one issue on which parents who have experienced this situation agree, it is that the manner in which they were informed was unsatisfactory.

Studies show that most parents are informed by a doctor[5]. In some cases parents are told separately of the news. Whichever parent is told first, he/she must wait for 'what seems like a lifetime' to share their thoughts and feelings with their partner.

The information provided also varies. Sometimes no details are given and at other times too much technical information is imparted too quickly to be fully taken in by the parents.

Grandparents and other family members will also want to know about the child's problems and may well be influential in determining how the family as a whole responds to the situation. Of course, there is a danger that one of the parents may be 'blamed' for what has happened and the question may well arise of whether subsequent children are likely to be affected.

As parents gradually come to terms with the news that their son or daughter has a learning disability they generally seek information and practical help to enable them to provide the best standard of care possible for their child. The assistance required by families caring for children with learning disabilities will vary depending on individual circumstances. Generally, however, parents of children with learning disabilities require the same advice and guidance as any parents. This might include information on changing, feeding, bathing and establishing sleeping routines. When parents ask direct questions about the extent and nature of their child's impairment it is best to be honest, but tactful.

What is especially important is that professionals are seen to share the worries and concerns. Whispered conversations in corridors and knowing glances between staff can add to the isolation and anxiety felt by parents. Technical jargon emphasises professional expertise but is unlikely to be helpful to parents.

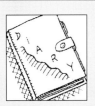

ACTIVITY 5
20 minutes
If you were the parent of a child with a learning disability what do you think would be the main questions which you would ask about your son or daughter's condition?

• Write down in your diary a list of four possible questions; for each question indicate whom you think would be the best person to provide an answer.

Many questions will have been generated from this Activity. You may have identified some which relate to the past (for example, 'Why did it happen?'); the present ('What can I do to help my child?'); or the future ('Will he or she be able to attend an ordinary school?'). Your list of people who would be able to answer these questions may have included a range of professionals.

Mathias[6] points out that it is only when informal sources prove inadequate that formal support services become involved, and outlines a hierarchy of types of support systems, ranging from informal to formal:

1. Natural help system (primarily kith-and-kin).
2. Mutual help system (self-help groups).
3. Non-professional help system (minister, priest or advice centre worker).

4. Professional help system (staff within health, social work and education services).

In this context, the function of formal helping agencies is to provide assistance and support which can supplement rather than replace the help that is provided informally. Commenting on the relationships which professionals establish with parents of children with Down syndrome, Byrne et al.[7] suggest: 'It is vital that professionals reassure and support parents and do nothing to undermine their feelings of competence and confidence even further by seeming to "take over".

Nurses involved in the provision of services for families with young children have an important role to play in helping parents develop the skills needed to care for a child with a disability. Most parents value the practical help they receive during the early days when they are coming to terms with their child's disability and appreciate the continuing support which nurses can offer within the framework of primary and community health care services.

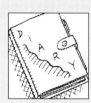

ACTIVITY 6
10 minutes
It is difficult to generalise about the effects on family relationships of caring for a child with a learning disability, as research findings are conflicting.

• Write down one or two factors which you think may help to strengthen relationships among family members and one or two factors which may adversely affect those relationships.

You may find that some of the factors which you have identified could apply to the care of any child. It is important to remember that families with a child with a learning disability are ordinary families who have to cope with additional problems.

The birth of a child can be a source of joy and pleasure. It can also lead to changes in lifestyle and relationships which result in stress and strain. There are often practical problems associated with looking after a child with a learning disability which means higher than usual childcare costs. Of course, lack of money is a major source of stress for any family.

Professionals are often the 'gatekeepers' to resources which can help families to cope with the additional costs of caring for a growing child with a learning disability. These additional costs may include:

• **Transport**
Extra journeys may be required to attend hospital and clinic appointments. If public transport is difficult to use, taxis can be an expensive alternative.

• **Incontinence**
Some children with learning disabilities are slow to learn to use the toilet. Soiled clothes need to be washed more often.

• **Food**
The child may require a special diet or special preparation of food.

• **Wear and tear of furniture and fittings**

In some instances, children with learning disabilities are hyperactive and can be destructive towards household items.

• **Special clothing requirements**

— Harder wearing garments will be required for children who are incontinent or who have a tendency to tear their clothes

— A child with an awkward gait will wear down shoes more quickly and wheelchairs can 'snag' clothes

— Parents' clothes may wear out more quickly through kneeling or playing on the floor with children who cannot walk.

• **Toys**

Children with learning disabilities may require additional stimulation. Parents may buy a variety of toys in order to keep their child's interest. These may also wear out quickly. Some areas have toy libraries which will help limit costs.

There are also 'hidden costs' involved in caring for a child with a learning disability. It is primarily women who provide care for people with disabilities who are living at home and, as Glendinning[8] comments, '...poverty, dependency and insecurity, in both the short and longer terms, will be the prices paid by women for their contribution to 'community care'.

Going to school

'When they were little, we were told to love them, they couldn't be educated. We had to sign that they couldn't be educated - we had to sign the education papers. It broke my heart. They said: "Just love them, give them as much love as you can", and you do. You make sure they don't burn themselves and other things like that. And then, when they grow older, we're "too protective"'[9].

This statement by a mother whose adult daughter has a learning disability poignantly illustrates the difficulties which arise for parents in the face of changing attitudes. It also highlights the fact that not so long ago children with learning disabilities were denied access to educational services if they were unable to attain a required standard.

The early 1980s legislation established that children have a right to an education which meets their individual needs. Subsequent legislation has amended the detail of the legislative framework, though the main provisions have remained unaltered since this time.

Currently, children and young people are considered to have 'special educational needs' if they have significantly greater difficulty in learning than most other children of their age; have a disability which prevents them from making effective use of educational facilities generally used by others of a similar age; are under the age of five years but will be likely to have a learning difficulty when over that age.

Education authorities thus have a duty to provide education for all children, but there is no obligation for children with learning difficulties to be educated in 'mainstream' schools[10]. Moreover, though the educational needs of children with learning disabilities under the age of five have to be ascertained, there is no requirement for education authorities to provide education until normal school age is reached. In relation to the standard of schooling, the law states only that the education provided for students with special educational needs must be 'adequate and efficient'.

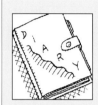

ACTIVITY 7
5 minutes
Suppose it was decided that the phrase 'adequate and efficient' should be replaced by a different form of words to determine the standard of education provided for students with special educational needs.

• What would you suggest?

Write down in your diary a possible alternative.

In writing your new phrase you might have included the word 'effective'. So, for example, you might advocate more effective provision for pre-school children. Clearly, this is important, because play is such a vital part of the development of all children. For a child with a learning disability it is especially important. Although all infants need love and attention and help to begin to explore their environment, a child with a learning disability has to rely heavily on others to create learning opportunities and stimulate interest.

From the age of two most children with learning disabilities have access to nursery school, nursery classes, day nurseries and play groups or other day care facilities where they have contact with non-disabled children.

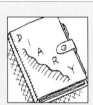

ACTIVITY 8
15 minutes
It is now common practice for disabled and non-disabled infants to mix within a single group.

Write down some of the potential benefits which might result from this arrangement and some of the potential problems.

You might have found conflicts and contradictions between your two lists. For example, in your lists of benefits you might have included providing the opportunity to be able to become a fully participating member of society. However, your 'problems list' might have included becoming seen as different and highlighting the disability.

In one study of children with Down syndrome[11], nearly all were able to attend a facility where they had contact with non-disabled children. Twenty eight per cent also attended a regular club or class, for example dancing lessons, sports club or Sunday school. For many children with learning disabilities, educational integration with non-disabled children will come to an end when they start school.

There has been considerable debate over the past 20 years about the pros and cons of integrated schooling. MacKay[12] comments:

'In part, this is because the right to equality of educational opportunity is often equated with identical educational provision for all pupils, and this is difficult to envisage in practice. Yet it is also recognised that segregated special education may be too sheltered an experience, too limited in its level of interest and challenge, and inadequate in preparing pupils for as full a life as possible in the community'.

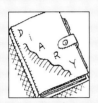

ACTIVITY 9
40 minutes
Imagine that you have been asked to join a working group which has been set up to plan the integration of children with severe learning disabilities within your local primary school. Each member of the group has been asked to prepare a short statement which outlines his/her personal view on the issue. Think what you would say in your statement and write down what this would be.

Most parents want their children to be happy. They want to hear the sound of laughter when their children are small. They want their children to have friends, to settle in school and to achieve all they can academically.

Starting school is a major step in everyone's life. The pain and pleasure involved is no different for a child with a learning disability. From the child's point of view, the things which make school good or bad are universal. School dinners, games, playtimes and whether the teacher shouts or not may seem far more important than the speed at which reading skills develop or how many numbers can be added together. At its best, school can provide an environment within which the child is able to develop his or her competence and confidence and which will provide a solid foundation for adult life.

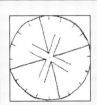

FOCUS
2 hours
• What services and facilities are available as resources for children with learning disabilities and their families who live near you?

• Do these resources encourage integration with non-disabled children or not?

• Discover as much as you can about local provision of health, social care and education services. Find out if there are any voluntary sector organisations or community groups active in the area. Is a local directory of services published?

There is no need to produce a lengthy report on services which are available but you should list the names of about 10 services/facilities, with a sentence or two to explain what each one offers. Include your findings in your community profile.

3. Becoming an adult

This Section focuses on the provision of services for adults with learning disabilities. Implications of the transition from childhood and adulthood are discussed and issues which arise in relation to continuing education, employment and leaving home are explored.

An inevitable transition?

Making the transition from childhood to adulthood is never a seamless process. Becoming an adult involves biological changes and the development of a new social identity.

Children and adults are normally viewed differently by people and are treated differently under the law. Jenkins[1] points out:

'There are the various thresholds of adulthood which are defined legally or administratively by the state. Crossed at different ages, these include criminal responsibility, sexual consent, the conditional or unconditional right to marry, the right to vote and the right to donate blood or organs for transplantation. Adulthood is in this sense bound up, in a weaker or stronger fashion, with citizenship. It is not, however, marked by a sharply defined change of legal status: there is, instead, an incremental inclusion into jural adulthood, culminating in Britain at the age of eighteen with the right to vote'.

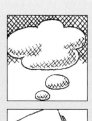

ACTIVITY 1
10 minutes
- At what age did you start to think of yourself as an adult?

- Looking back, can you remember a specific point in your life at which you thought 'I'm no longer a child'?

- Do you still think that this is the point at which the transition took place?

- Write down in your diary brief responses to these questions.

Jenkins suggests that the transition from childhood to adulthood is neither inevitable nor natural. Rather, it is something which is determined by people within a society — it is socially constructed.

For someone with a learning disability, being treated as an 'eternal child' can create an effective barrier to adulthood. Having a learning disability does not in itself disempower someone from voting if he or she is over the age of 18 years, or prevent someone of legal age from getting married.

On these matters, the law is based on judging whether or not an individual has sufficient understanding of the consequences of his or her actions. Someone with a learning disability may be considered to have sufficient insight to get married. You may think that a good case could be made for the view that *no one* has sufficient understanding of the consequences of his or her actions to be allowed to enter into a 'till death us do part' marriage contract! It all depends on what is meant by 'sufficient' understanding or insight. It is worth remembering that not so long ago women were considered to have insufficient insight to be allowed to vote.

Of course, having insight is not something which is present or absent. There can be degrees of insight. In the following extract, Lea[2] presents an analysis of comments made by two people living in an institution which she interprets as showing awareness of environment and as having views on and likes and dislikes.

•In the morning I get up at 5 o'clock to make my bed and wash my face and clean my teeth and sweep my room and have a bath and brush my hair. The bell rings for breakfast and I go to work at eight in the morning. I am busy with a mat. For lunch I ate [corn on the cob] at twelve o'clock. And then I go to work at one o'clock and I would like to read and do drawings.
(Dorothy, aged 42)•

•In the morning we get up 5 o'clock and then we dress [a more disabled resident] in the morning and I feed her. At 9 o'clock we go to handicraft and at 1 o'clock we go back to the handicraft until 4 o'clock. And at night-time I have a nice sleep and then I have nice dreams about the group and the nice time we have there. I look forward to it all week because I like it very much.
(Margie, aged 45)•

•Both Dorothy and Margie, while documenting the routine of life in the institution, also comment on what gives them enjoyment. These pieces clearly convey that their lives revolve around work, with very little time for recreation or pleasurable pursuits... These extracts illustrate that people regarded as mentally less competent do have insight into their current circumstances, and can communicate this effectively and efficiently. Certainly to describe the writers of these pieces as lacking insight or as being incapable of expressing themselves would be to do them a grave disservice.•

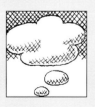

ACTIVITY 2
20 minutes
How would you feel if you were not allowed to take responsibility for your own actions? Think about ways in which you are treated as 'a responsible adult' and write down what some of the implications would be if this ended?

Adulthood is associated with legal rights and social responsibilities. Adults have scope to take decisions which affect themselves and to exercise choice over how they live. Entering adulthood is often a turbulent time in which we are determined to change our relationship with the world. Teenagers tend to emphasise the differences between themselves and the previous generation. They often seek to create allegiances with groups of like-minded people. Adolescence can involve trying out new things and making mistakes. For parents this can be a worrying time: after a period of relative stability during childhood a whole new set of problems and difficulties may begin to emerge.

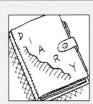

ACTIVITY 3
30 minutes
For many parents the worst fears for their son or daughter are probably that they will take 'hard' drugs; be exploited sexually; become involved in criminal activities; be subjected to violence.

- If the parents of a non-disabled 16-year-old were to ask your opinion on how they should handle one of these situations, what advice would you give?

- Would your advice be different if the 16-year-old has a learning disability?

- Write down brief comments.

For parents of young people with learning disabilities there can be additional anxieties, based on legitimate concerns about the person's vulnerability and lack of opportunities for continuing personal development. In a study of the views of young people with learning disabilities and their parents, McConkey[3] found that there was most discrepancy when it came to their hopes and ambitions for the future. When asked about what job they would like in the future most of the young people were able to give one or more preferences. Unlike their parents' focus on special services they wanted to have an ordinary occupation. None of the students envisaged attending a long-term day centre.

McConkey comments: '...the students mentioned a range of jobs, many of which would be unrealistic but equally a significant minority of parents do see possibilities for jobs for which they feel their son or daughter could be capable. What are services and parents doing to help make this a reality at least for some?'

In a study of services for mothers caring for children with learning disabilities, one woman's feelings about her daughter's transition from school to a centre for adults is reported[4]:

'It just didn't work for Lisa. Lisa was placed with adults. It broke my heart, because even though she was 16, to me she was a child. In the centre they were all jealous of her because there were a lot of older people with different handicaps. They used to knock her about. She was in hospital twice and in the end I took her out of the centre altogether. Your problems start then because you know you can't cope with them at home all the time'.

Continuing education and employment

As you will have discovered, people with learning disabilities are not an homogenous group. All religious and ethnic backgrounds are represented, although service providers do not always acknowledge that this is the case[5,6]. Furthermore, there is as great a range of 'personality types' as in the population as a whole and individuals' interests cover a wide spread of social and cultural activities.

The nature and extent of people's learning disabilities also encompass considerable variation. The adjectives 'mild', 'moderate', 'severe' and 'profound' are sometimes used to describe different levels of severity of an individual's learning disability. It has been argued that just as school authorities are required to take account of an individual's particular educational needs, so, too, should post-school services. Unfortunately, continuing education services and vocational training opportunities are still few and far between for people with learning disabilities.

There are many examples of people with moderate or mild learning disabilities holding down jobs within manufacturing and service industries, although at times of high unemployment this becomes much less common.

The advantages of work are the same for people with learning disabilities as they are for everyone else. Having a job promotes a feeling of personal worth and value to the community. Mixing with colleagues can provide companionship and impart a sense of belonging. Going to work provides a structure to the day and week, and can also provide a sense of purpose. Lastly, work provides financial rewards which offer people increased choice as consumers.

Of course, there are also disadvantages associated with being an employee — not everyone experiences work as a positive part of life and for someone with a learning disability there is an increased danger of exploitation by an unscrupulous employer.

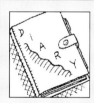

ACTIVITY 4
10 minutes
How important is work?

* Think about how important work is to you and consider the views on work of people you know.

* Write down your opinion on whether or not emphasis should be placed on enabling people with learning disabilities to find jobs.

The importance assigned to work in people's lives will vary greatly. Some may regard work as a 'necessary evil', while others may view it as essential for personal development and fulfilment. Some people will be happy with the balance that they have achieved between time spent at work and the pursuit of other activities while others will resent the amount of time that is taken up by work. For most people, however, there is some flexibility in deciding how much time to devote to earning money.

The bulk of current post-school provision for people with all levels of learning disabilities involves day care services. These services usually offer group-based activities and little or no chance to earn money. In reviewing the literature on day care services for adults, Brearley and Mandelstam[7] highlight the following issues:

- They are usually provided as part of a package of health and social services which often lack cohesive overall strategic planning

- They are often seen as a substitute for other services, especially hospital or residential care, and as a cheaper alternative

- There is a debate about the extent to which such services should focus on care (rehabilitation, respite, therapy, etc) or on services which enable and empower (education, employment, leisure, etc)

- Care tends to be seen as related to centre-based provision but this is not necessarily so. There is further debate about the extent to which services should be based in centres (buildings) or incorporate a wide range of community facilities which may or may not be based in buildings.

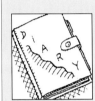

ACTIVITY 5
30 minutes
It has been argued that the best way to determine how day care centres develop in the future would be to enable service-users to have a say in how they are run.

- Think how service-users could be involved in the management of a centre and write down possible steps which could be taken to achieve this.

There are many ways in which service-users can be given more of a say in the running of services. Whittaker et al.[8] describe the background to the establishment of a London office for People First, an organisation which is run by people with learning disabilities to promote and develop self-advocacy, and comment:

'A first step was to make sure that People First members were involved at every stage of setting up the office. Adaptations and alterations to conventional ways of doing things were necessary at various points to enable this to happen. A simple but important example was writing the job application form in language which everyone could understand. In working out the job descriptions, the qualities and skills needed by the workers, the questions to be asked during the interviewing, it was People First members' ideas which took priority[9].

It may be, of course, that service-users do not want to be 'placed' in a day centre. Within this context it is argued that people with learning disabilities should be given more control over how they spend their time. Increasingly, the development of 'service brokerage' arrangements is being seen as a way of ensuring that each service-user is offered an appropriate mix of work, leisure and educational opportunities.

This issue of service brokerage, whereby an individual with care and support requirements is able to draw on the expertise of an independent broker to put together an individually-tailored package of services, is considered further in Section 4.

An encouraging development in recent years has been an increase in the extent to which further education colleges are catering for students with learning disabilities. From the point of view of many young people with learning disabilities, the opportunity to attend college provides an attractive alternative to attending a 'day care centre' or an 'adult training centre'. Like everyone else, people with learning disabilities are able to benefit from education throughout their lives. It has been pointed out that in our society the general principle seems to be that the better you are at learning the more educational assistance you will receive. A case of 'those with least need get most'!

Independence or interdependence?

Professionals working with people with learning disabilities often stress that their intention is that clients should 'develop new skills'. Moreover, it is often recommended that the effectiveness of services should be measured by how much progress individuals have made in learning self-help skills.

The title of a book by Carr and Collins[9], which offers 'a practical guide to teaching people with learning disabilities', is *Working Towards Independence*. Growth and development throughout a person's lifetime is often characterised as a process which involves moving from a state of dependence in childhood to independence in adulthood and, in old age, a return to a state of dependence. Adulthood as a state of 'independence from being cared for', as implied in this process is, for some people with continuing and complex health and social care requirements, neither a desirable nor an attainable goal. If adoption of this approach extends beyond formal education settings to impact on an individual's home life, it may result in the person's becoming socially isolated.

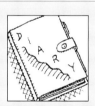

ACTIVITY 6
20 minutes
Loneliness is a major problem in the lives of many adults with learning disabilities — even for those who are living with other people.

• Think of some of the ways in which non-disabled people combat loneliness and write down the extent to which these strategies could be adopted by people with learning disabilities.

People generally combat loneliness by establishing contact with others in whom they are interested and who are interested in them. For people with learning disabilities, there is a danger that becoming more independent will mean spending less time with those people who are interested in them. Moreover, having a learning disability often means that an individual has to work harder and is less skilled in establishing the sort of personal friendship and acquaintanceship network which can prevent social isolation.

An alternative way of conceptualising changes which occur during the lifetime of an individual is as shifting patterns of inter-dependence. As children grow, the focus of their social activities generally begins to broaden to include people from outside the family. Friendships develop and take on more significance — particularly during the teenage years.

Intimate relationships are formed with people outside the family. Getting a job entails the establishment of relationships with others which are based on mutual economic advantage. People very often move from the family home to live with friends or with a partner. Even when someone chooses to live alone he or she normally develops a network of friends, colleagues and acquaintances which involves mutually supportive relationships. Unless we lead a very austere existence, we learn how other people live by means of newspapers, television and radio. Very few of us, therefore, could claim to live a life that is truly independent of others.

Supported living options

In view of the standards of care which have been deemed acceptable for people with learning disabilities in the past it is perhaps not surprising that parents often express concern about the future.

MacLachlan et al.[10] articulate the feelings of mothers of people with learning disabilities, and outline the sort of service they would like:

'We know that the time for permanent care will come, and that it will leave a strangeness and emptiness within us. We in no way wish to relinquish totally our responsibility and would like to retain some control both from the medical and caring points of view. We believe that residential care must be provided within the community and not in the "wilds". In this way people with handicaps can continue to be part of the community, and local residents can perhaps in some way monitor what happens to them. Care must be taken to see that things remain familiar, consistent and, above all, comfortable and cheerful'.

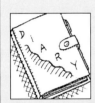

ACTIVITY 7
30 minutes
When a young person with a learning disability leaves the family home, what do you consider to be the most important features of that person's future place of residence?

Think about your own home life and the sorts of additional help which someone with a learning disability might require. Write down a list of the things which you feel would contribute to 'quality'.

Perhaps the most important factor contributing to the quality of life for the person with a learning disability living away from home, is the level and nature of support which he/she receives from family, friends and professionals. For this reason, people often choose to live in staffed residential homes as tenants.

Adults with learning disabilities have the same right as anyone else to move from the family home if they wish. Parents also realise that as they grow older they will be less able to provide the necessary care and support and that, after their death their son or daughter will still require help. Leaving home means that parents are often able to assist in smoothing the transition and that they can continue to play an active part in the life of their son or daughter.

People with learning disabilities experience the sense of loss associated with the death of a parent as much as anyone else[11]. The establishment of a stable and supportive environment prior to this event can help the individual when bereavement occurs.

The creation of small, community-based residential homes does not mean that integration will be achieved, or that institutionalisation will be avoided[12]. Nevertheless, in many areas there are well-established examples of good quality domiciliary and residential care services for people with learning disabilities. Unfortunately, these are insufficient to meet current requirements, for in addition to people leaving their family homes, the planned discharge of people who have been inappropriately living in long-stay hospitals has added to the demand for these small, community-based residential homes.

Current thinking suggests that rather than having 'hospitals', 'hostels', 'group homes' or even 'supported accommodation', for people with learning disabilities, they require access to a range of ordinary housing options with the guarantee of continuing support at a level which is commensurate with high-quality, individualised care. Normally this is called supported living.

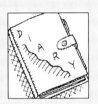

ACTIVITY 8
20 minutes
The relationship between an individual and the place in which he or she is staying is summarised by various titles: prison inmate; hospital patient; hostel resident; housing association tenant.

• Think about the status which is associated with each of these titles and the extent to which the holder of each title will have control over his or her surroundings. Note your comments in your diary.

The traditional approach to developing residential services for people with learning disabilities is based on:

• Grouping people together because they happen to have similar types of disabilities
• Judging the effectiveness of services by the extent to which the service-user's skills increase
• Requiring people to achieve a pre-determined level of functioning to demonstrate that they are ready to move on to some other form of accommodation
• Assuming that service-users are not able to determine their own needs or exercise real control over their own lives.

Supported living has evolved as an alternative, more imaginative approach to solving the problems experienced by people needing high levels of support for the activities of daily living. Rather than assessing people for the purpose of 'placement', service-providers who wish to create supported living options focus on the establishment of individually relevant and valued patterns of care and support. Among other things this means that each service-user should be entitled to: live in a home of his/her own; be able to exercise choice over whether or not to live with anyone else; receive the quantity and quality of support which is necessary to meet his/her requirements.

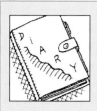

You may have identified more disadvantages than advantages. An important aspect of supported living is that the individual's views and preferences should be taken into account. Being *required* to share a bedroom (or even a home) with one or more people means that this is not happening.

The fundamental principle of successful supported living schemes is that the costs of each person's housing, daily living expenses and support requirements should be met in full from budgets intended for each of these purposes. An individual's housing costs should be met by housing benefit or mortgage assistance; daily living costs should be met by benefits and allowances; and support requirements should be funded by the appropriate social care and health agencies.

In some cases an individual may also be entitled to receive money from the Independent Living Fund, which is a discretionary allowance intended to enable very severely disabled people to pay for domiciliary care which will allow them to stay in their own homes.

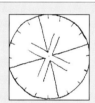

FOCUS
2 hours
Values Into Action (VIA) is a national organisation which campaigns with people who have learning difficulties* to end 'the injustice and misunderstanding which have impoverished the lives of people with learning difficulties'.

VIA believes that all people with learning difficulties:

- Have the same rights as other people, and should be allowed the same choices
- Are just as important as other people, and should be treated with dignity and respect
- Can live in the same way and in the same places as other people live, and should be given the help they need to make this possible
- Should be allowed and, where necessary, helped to have the same opportunities in schools, colleges, work and leisure as other people.

The nursing profession has also issued statements of beliefs which underpin quality and effective nursing care.

- In about 1,000 words compare VIA's statement with a statement of beliefs made by nurses and discuss the implications for the provision of health services for people with learning disabilities.

* VIA prefers to use the term 'learning difficulties' rather than 'learning disability'

4. Creating healthy services

In this Section we explore some of the issues involved in the development of effective health services for people with learning disabilities and their families. We look at changes in the ways in which services are co-ordinated, the contribution of health-care professionals to service provision, and health problems commonly associated with learning disabilities. We also highlight some challenges for the future.

All pulling together?

Over the past 25 years there have been marked changes in the structure and organisational framework of services for people with learning disabilities and their families. From a situation whereby 'receiving specialist services' was largely synonymous with 'admission to hospital', and specialist services were provided almost exclusively by medical and nursing staff, a *multi-agency approach* has gradually evolved. Social care, education and housing agencies, voluntary sector organisations, community groups and the private sector now have major roles to play.

During the 1970s the term 'community care' was normally used to indicate something other than long-stay hospital care. The creation of hostels for people with learning disabilities was considered an appropriate way of providing community care.

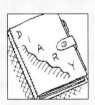

ACTIVITY 1
45 minutes
• What do you think is meant by the term 'community care'?

• Now look at how the term is defined in recent government documents and note in your diary your thoughts on the extent to which this differs from 'something other than long-stay hospital care'.

Changed attitudes towards long-stay hospital provisions is, in part, the result of the development of the multi-agency approach. Instead of being seen as 'the answer', hospitals are now regarded as having been part of the problem for people with learning disabilities.

As the notion that people with learning disabilities should be admitted for long-term care to large, isolated, specialist hospitals was rejected during the 1970s, there was growing recognition that new forms of domiciliary support, residential care and day services would be required. Since then, the need for collaboration among agencies to provide a co-ordinated and comprehensive range of local services for people with learning disabilities and their families has been a recurrent theme in relation to policy formation and the planning, management and provision of services.

Even within the framework of health service provision the involvement of a variety of professionals is now considered to be necessary for the establishment of a *multidisciplinary approach*. Contemporary specialist health care services for people with learning disabilities normally include speech and language therapy, clinical psychology, physiotherapy and occupational therapy. The services of art, drama and music therapists and other members of professions allied to medicine may also be available.

Nurses with specialist qualifications in working with people with learning disabilities have continued to play an important role in the provision of services. It has very often been specialist community nurses who have led the development of local, community-based alternatives to long-stay hospital provision: 'Through their daily work with clients and their families community nurses will identify areas of need within the community. Part of their responsibility is to provide a comprehensive report to managers of areas of service where change is required'[1].

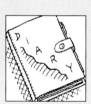

ACTIVITY 2
10 minutes
The Cullen Report[2], on the nursing needs of people with learning disabilities included the observation that the skills of specialist nurses working with people with learning disabilities are 'facility-independent'.

* Do you think that this statement could apply to all nurses? Write down the extent to which you consider this to be the case.

During the 1980s there was considerable regional variation in the development of services which could offer individuals and families a framework of co-ordinated support and assistance. Despite the absence of joint planning arrangements at a strategic level, joint NHS and local authority 'community teams' (usually called community mental handicap teams, or CMHTs) were established to co-ordinate the planning of services at a local level.

A survey carried out at the beginning of the 1980s identified 71 CMHTs throughout Britain[3] whereas a similar survey carried out in England during 1987/88[4] identified 348 teams.

Highlighting the existence of a wide range of operational models, Griffiths and Brown[4] pointed out that there are questions about the different sizes of teams and the different populations they cover:

'Teams with more than 20 members will operate in markedly different ways to smaller teams. Teams covering populations of fewer than 60,000 may be expected to have different operational policies from teams covering 120,000 or more people'.

In charting the 'natural history' of this approach to co-ordinating services, Mansell[5] comments:

'...it may be that the community mental handicap team is, like the 25-place residential unit, a transitional phase in service development, the main contribution of which is to focus attention in the right place and get people to ask pertinent questions about service delivery'.

The Audit Commission for Local Authorities in England and Wales, in its influential report on community care[6], noted the positive contribution which community mental handicap teams could make to successful community care schemes but also pointed out that developments of this sort amounted to '... a radical departure from the generally accepted ways of doing things at present in the NHS and within local government'.

The Audit Commission report concluded that slow and uneven progress towards community care was due to fundamental underlying problems. Its analysis included the observation:

'A fragmented organisation structure causes delays and difficulties; and there has been a failure to adapt systems and structures to accommodate the shift in policy'.

How best to overcome the difficulties which arise when agencies and organisations are required to work together to create effective community care services has been addressed in various ways in the Griffiths Report[7], in the Government White Paper, *Caring for People*[8] and in the subsequent NHS and Community Care Act 1990.

The NHS and Community Care Act 1990 was not fully implemented until April 1993. Among other things, the Act requires local authorities and health authorities to publish community care plans which outline how they intend to develop services for particular groups of people, including people with learning disabilities and their families. Some community care plans are prepared and published jointly by NHS and local authority staff as a single document. In other instances separate documents are produced.

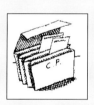

ACTIVITY 3
5 minutes
Write down brief comments on one problem which you feel would arise in preparing a joint NHS and local authority plan in your area. Include your notes in your community profile.

Problems may arise because of simple administrative differences (for example, boundaries not being co-terminous), or it may be that there are different organisational priorities. In some parts of the country health, social care and housing agencies work well together. In other parts there is little or no collaboration.

Particular health problems

Within the framework of the NHS and Community Care Act, local authorities have 'lead agency' responsibility for co-ordinating the provision of services for people with learning disabilities and their families. Specialist health-care professionals are now able to concentrate their efforts on helping to improve the health and well-being of service- users.

There are many health deficits and medical problems associated with learning disabilities which can be dealt with properly only if adequate time and professional expertise is available. Some health-related problems may be addressed by professionals who do not specialise in working with people with learning disabilities. In other instances, however, specialist expertise and experience in the area is required as a foundation for effective care. Furthermore, many people with disability themselves, as well as their carers, will be unable to recognise the significance of physical symptoms. The health of many people with learning disabilities is therefore not always all that it should be[9]. Sines identifies particular problems which can be experienced by people with learning disabilities. He noted that there are:

- Those who have an identified and diagnosed mental illness which is susceptible to treatment

- Those whose behaviour has been identified as challenging, disruptive or antisocial and for whom specific support services are required

- Those who have an associated physical illness which requires ongoing skilled nursing care and support, for example people with chronic epilepsy or chronic respiratory disorders

- Those who have additional physical or sensory handicaps which require nursing and medical care

- Those who require intensive nursing support to compensate for lower levels of ability and self-help skills

- Older people who have additional nursing and medical needs.

In addition it is known that there is a high incidence of Alzheimer's disease in people with Down syndrome.

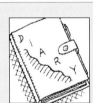

ACTIVITY 4
20 minutes
People with learning disabilities experience the same health problems as anyone else.

- Think of a service in which you have worked and write down the problems which staff would be likely to experience if a person with a learning disability were to be admitted or referred. It may be that this has happened, in which case you will be able to relate first-hand experience.

Generally, the main difficulty experienced by staff is associated with communication. Someone with a learning disability may not understand instructions or requests and may be unable to provide necessary information. This can lead to anxiety for the person using the service and can be frustrating for staff. For these reasons it is often necessary to allow more time to communicate with someone with a learning disability and to encourage the person to involve a representative, supporter or advocate.

There is a wide range of NHS services which provide support and treatment for conditions associated with learning disabilities or which aim to limit the effects on the individual and family. For instance, primary health care services, and in particular public health nurses (health visitors), play an important role in screening children to detect the presence of conditions or disorders which can lead to a learning disability.

An example of this is the routine testing of all babies to detect the presence of phenylketonuria. If undetected, this metabolic disorder will result in damage to the developing child's central nervous system. However, the condition is easily detected by administration of a test which involves collecting a small sample of the baby's blood. Children who have this condition require a special diet to avoid impairment of their ability to learn.

Routine developmental assessments can help to identify children whose development is delayed. Early identification of learning difficulties allows further investigations to be carried out to establish causal factors and can enable early assistance if required. Other measures which can be taken to reduce the incidence of learning disability later include the immunisation of girls to prevent the possibility of their contracting rubella during pregnancy.

People with learning disabilities can have particular health problems. Someone with a learning disability who has a communication problem may be unable to tell others that he or she is experiencing pain or feeling unwell. Often a carer who knows the person well will suspect that 'something is wrong' but will be uncertain of the nature of the medical problem. For this reason routine health checks are important.

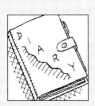

ACTIVITY 5
20 minutes
Think about a person with a learning disability with whom you have been working, and note down whether or not that person has any health problems.

• How might you do this in a systematic manner?

• What tests would be required to be carried out to find out more about the person's current health status?

Epilepsy is much more common among people with learning disabilities than in the general population and its prevalence increases directly with the severity of the person's learning disability. Many people who have a learning disability also have impaired mobility. Sensory loss is also common. For someone with Down syndrome there is a 50% likelihood that he or she will have a congenital heart disorder, and dementia-type changes are frequent in people with Down syndrome over the age of 40.

An additional health risk for people with a learning disability is that they have an increased likelihood of contracting hepatitis B. The occurrence of this condition has been more common in long-stay hospitals than in the population as a whole. For this reason universal vaccination is recommended for people with learning disabilities who are moving into shared home accommodation and for staff who are working in these settings.

A small proportion of people with learning disabilities exhibit behaviour which is particularly challenging for service providers[10]. The sorts of behaviours involved can range from destruction of clothes and belongings to self-injury or verbal and physical aggression towards others.

In the past it has been common practice to group together people with challenging behaviour. Current thinking, however, is that if an individual's behaviour is dangerous to others, this is primarily an argument for well-organised staff support and, in extreme cases, for one-person placement.

A small number of people with learning disabilities need to be detained in hospital (or an equivalent setting) because of their behaviour. This sort of action is not undertaken lightly. It is very much a 'last resort' and requires that the correct legal processes be followed.

A few people with learning disabilities become offenders and enter the prison system. A review of health and social services for mentally disordered offenders[11], which included consideration of people with learning disabilities, commented: '...we consider that, for prisoners who need them, there should be access to all the necessary health and social services, such as education. In some cases diversion to health and social services may need to be considered: for example, if the person is clearly vulnerable or subjected to victimisation'.

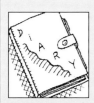

ACTIVITY 6
20 minutes
In view of their vulnerability, and the higher-than-average incidence of sexual abuse which is experienced by people with learning disabilities, it has been suggested that sex education is a priority for this group.

• What do you consider would be the principal objections to the introduction of a comprehensive sex education programme for teenagers with learning disabilities?

• Make a list of the main objections which you would expect to be raised and comment on the validity of each.

The question of sex education often provokes strong reactions. Some people consider it necessary to ensure that young people are as fully informed as possible about all the issues while others feel that greater knowledge can be dangerous.

People with learning disabilities are certainly vulnerable to exploitation and abuse. However, it is recognised that having a learning disability should not deny a person the opportunity to develop an intimate relationship if she or he so chooses. The objections to the introduction of a sex education programme for people with learning disabilities are generally the same as those raised in relation to sex education for other young people. The rationale for developing such a programme would also apply generally.

Raising awareness, expectations and standards

Public awareness of the difficulties faced by people with learning disabilities will vary depending on individual experiences and level of interest. Increased awareness can lead to greater understanding and the removal of barriers to integration. People with learning disabilities need other people to include them in community life.

Awareness can be a double-edged sword, however. People who are aware that someone with a learning disability is moving into the neighbourhood may (and very often do) object. Often, their objections are based on their lack of awareness about disability. They might also have a prejudiced attitude about living alongside anyone who is not like them. At a time when people are being discharged from long-stay hospital settings to live in ordinary houses, this can pose considerable problems. Reporting on the resettlement of people with learning disabilities Collins[12] highlights two different approaches which health-care professionals can take when confronted with this situation:

'Some resettlement programmes have a policy of talking to potential neighbours at a very early stage in order to defuse problems from the beginning. This, in fact, they are required to do following a ruling by the Health Service Commissioner that health authority staff are failing in their duty if they do not consult with neighbours prior to opening a community house'.

'I came across two areas where, after adhering to this direction, the potential house-vendor had been intimidated by neighbours into withdrawing from the sale. Three other health authorities I visited deliberately took the position that there was no issue to be discussed. Managers in these authorities believed that notifying prospective neighbours of the proposed use of the house, and holding meetings supposedly to allay fears, merely served to provide a forum for trouble: it suggested to people that they had cause for concern. One manager refused to attend meetings called by prospective neighbours because he refused to provide them with "a forum in which to air their prejudices". If you refuse to listen to people's complaints, he said, there is nothing they can do'.

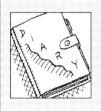

ACTIVITY 7
10 minutes
Of the two approaches outlined above which do you think is better? Write down your opinion and a brief explanation.

The question of whether or not neighbours should be consulted about plans for people with learning disabilities to be housed within a particular community often elicits strong opinions. On the one hand it is argued that there are advantages to be gained in involving members of the community at an early stage — social integration cannot be achieved if neighbours do not play an active part in making newcomers feel welcome. On the other hand, it is argued that as it is not common practice to tell neighbours about yourself when moving into an area, people with learning disabilities should not be treated differently.

Public awareness and knowledge about the problems experienced by people with learning disabilities is generally very limited. Clearly, much work needs to be done to educate and inform people about the issues involved. It is likely, however, that as the approach to service delivery moves away from segregation, members of the general public will become more comfortable with the idea of belonging to an inclusive local community.

As we saw with public awareness, there is more than one side to be considered in relation to raising expectations. On the one hand, families who are providing care and support for someone with a learning disability need to be encouraged to adopt a 'realistic' outlook. There is certainly no point in health-care professionals, or others, encouraging unrealistic expectations for the future treatment or care of their son or daughter. It cannot help parents to have their hopes raised that something dramatic can happen, just to have them dashed when the expected 'miracle' does not occur.

On the other hand, parent power has been instrumental in improving practices and creating a wide range of innovative caring services for people with learning disabilities. Parents who have experienced the availability of school education for their sons or daughters are less likely to accept the piecemeal approach to post-school provision which is too often the norm. Nurses can assist the process of raising expectations by supporting parents in their fight for better services.

Of course, it is not only parents who can have raised expectations. People with learning disabilities have been treated as powerless — largely because they are powerless within the present system. Individual service-users are often excluded from discussions about plans for their own futures and generally have little say in the sorts of services which they receive.

Perhaps the most obvious way in which this could change is by modifying the way in which the care management process operates. In current community care arrangements, the responsibility for allocating social care resources rests with a care manager, acting on behalf of the local authority. The care manager determines an individual's 'needs' through a process of 'assessment' and then will decide on a 'package of care'.

An alternative approach, which is gaining support, is to replace the care management system with one based on 'service brokerage'. In this approach, service-users should receive money with which to purchase services that they, in collaboration with others, consider best able to meet their own needs. A 'service broker' then acts as a representative of the service-user to negotiate and purchase a 'package of care'. This system has the distinct advantage that it gives real power (purchasing power) to the service-user[13].

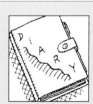

ACTIVITY 8
30 minutes
The NHS and Community Care Act 1990 established a separation between 'purchasers or commissioners' of services and 'providers' in relation to both health and social care. In the case of service brokerage the service-user becomes 'the purchaser'.

• Write down a list of advantages of a service-user with a learning disability being the purchaser of his/her own care and support services. Note some of the difficulties which might arise.

A study by Zarb and Nadash[14] found that disabled people who receive payments to allow them to make their own arrangements for personal and domestic assistance almost invariably express greater satisfaction with their support arrangements and their reliability than those using allocated services. In addition, people using 'payment schemes' were able to put together more cost-effective packages of care and support. Support arrangements financed through payment schemes were, on average, 30-40% cheaper than equivalent service-based support.

However, an in-depth evaluation of an Independent Living Project[15] has highlighted some of the difficulties which can arise in relation to the employment of personal assistants by disabled people:

- Personal assistants working in the home of their employer are not afforded the same legal protection as employees in almost every other occupation

- Many disabled people require support to enable them to employ personal assistants, for example, in dealing with insurance and medical issues and in the initial self-assessment of their requirements

- Unsuitable housing, lack of adaptations or a shortage of nursing and physiotherapy services may lead to personal assistants undertaking additional tasks which, arguably, are outside their remit and which raise issues about the appropriate source of funding for such tasks.

How to raise standards

We conclude this module with a brief look at how best to raise standards of care for people with learning disabilities and their families. From an historical point of view much has been gained. 'Warehousing' of people with learning disabilities is no longer considered to be an acceptable way of treating people whose only 'crime' is to have an impaired ability to learn. Specialist health-care services in general, and specialist community nursing services in particular, have been directly involved in a social revolution which has transformed the future outlook for many people with learning disabilities. The challenge must now be taken up by non-specialist service providers and individual citizens. The concept of 'inclusion' should become the driving force in the coming years.

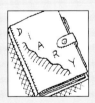

ACTIVITY 9
20 minutes
- What steps can be taken to include people with learning disabilities in ordinary community activities?

- Think about a club or leisure facility which you attend fairly regularly. What would be the reaction of others if a person with a learning disability attended? Does this already happen?

- Write down your thoughts on how someone with a learning disability could be included in this activity.

There is no reason why people with learning disabilities should not use the same facilities and enjoy the same activities as others, although to do so they often need to be encouraged and supported.

One positive example of what can be achieved was expressed by four people with learning disabilities living in a staffed house who were invited to join a local bowling club. Having met one of the residents, who indicated that she could not play bowls but would like to learn, the club secretary consulted with members of the club and arranged for lessons to be offered to all four residents. All are now full members of the club, which not only enables them to have regular physical exercise but also means that they have made new friends and have become part of their local community.

Conclusion

For people with learning disabilities to be included as full members of society, systems and procedures need to be established to provide homes, meaningful activities, care and support. What is also required is the commitment and strength of people who are not willing to stand back and allow those who are vulnerable and disadvantaged to face continuing discrimination and ill-treatment.

Nurses are well-placed to influence standards of care for people with learning disabilities and their families — both in relation to the way in which they are treated when they come into contact with nursing services and in how they are treated within society as a whole.

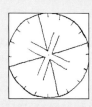

FOCUS
2–3 hours
- Find out the opinions of a parent with a son or daughter who has a learning disability, on the past, present and future of services.

- Make contact with a parent of someone who has a learning disability and explain that you wish to interview him or her as part of a project which you are undertaking.

- Before you interview the person think about some of the questions which you might wish to ask. The aim is to find out the person's opinions on the standard of services which his or her son or daughter has received in the past, is currently receiving, and which the parent would like to see available in the future.

- Ensure that any questions that you ask are phrased sensitively (we have seen how important language is) and allow the person to answer in his or her own way. Take notes, unless the person who is being interviewed objects. If note-taking is not possible, write down the main points which were raised during the interview immediately afterwards.

Write a report on the opinions expressed by the person interviewed (1,000 words maximum).

References

PART 1: MENTAL HEALTH

1. What is mental health?

1   World Health Organisation. Basic documents: preamble to the constitution of the World Health Organisation. In: Gillan, R. *Philosophical Medical Ethics.* Chichester: Wiley, 1986.
2   Sedgwick, P. Illness — mental and otherwise. In: Edwards, R. B. (ed) *Psychiatry and Ethics.* New York: Prometheus, 1982.
3   American Psychiatric Association. *Diagnostic and Statistical Manual of Mental Disorders* (3rd edn). *DSMIII.* Washington DC: American Psychiatric Association, 1980.
4   Szasz, T. S. *Ideology and Insanity.* New York: Doubleday, 1970.
5   Wright, H., Giddey, M. *Mental Health Nursing. From first principles to professional practice.* London: Chapman & Hall, 1993.

2. The importance of self-awareness

1   Bond, M. *Stress amd Self-awareness: A guide for nurses.* London: Heinemann, 1986.
2   Brill, N.I. *Working with People: The helping process* (4th edition). London: Longman, 1990.
3   Burnard, P. *Learning Human Skills: A guide for nurses.* London: Heinemann, 1985.
4   Stockwell, F. *The Unpopular Patient.* London: Royal College of Nursing, 1972.
5   Rogers, C. *On Becoming a Person.* London: Constable, 1974.

4. Professional aspects of mental health nursing

1   Griffiths, R. *Community Care: Agenda for Action.* A Report to the Secretary of State for Social Services. London: HMSO, 1988.
2   National Health Service Review. *Working for Patients.* Command Paper 555. London: HMSO, 1989.
3   Department of Health, Department of Social Security, Welsh Office, Scottish Office. *Caring for People: Community care in the next decade and beyond.* London: HMSO, 1989. Command Paper 849.
4   Ory, M. G., Bond, K. (eds). *Ageing and Health Care.* London: Routledge, 1989.
5   Gearing, B., Johnson, M., Heller, T. *Mental Health Problems in Old Age: A reader.* Chichester: Wiley, 1989.
6   Lavender, A., Holloway, F. (eds). *Community Care in Practice: Services for the continuing care client.* Chichester: Wiley, 1988.
7   Barton, R. *Institutional Neurosis* (3rd edn). Bristol: Wright, 1976.
8   Goffman, E. *Asylums.* Harmondsworth: Penguin, 1961 (Reprinted 1987).
9   Heywood Jones, I. *Helping Hands.* London: Macmillan Education, 1989.
10   Killen, S. In: Wright, H., Giddey, M. *Mental Health Nursing. From first principles to professional practice.* London: Chapman & Hall, 1993.
11   United Kingdom Central Council for Nursing, Midwifery and Health Visiting. *Project 2000. A new preparation for practice.* London: UKCC, 1986.
12   United Kingdom Central Council for Nursing, Midwifery and Health visiting. *Project 2000. Professional Paper 9: The Final Proposals.* London: UKCC, 1987.
13   Stuart, G.W., Sundeen, S.J. *Principles and Practice of Psychiatric Nursing.* London: C.V. Mosby Co., 1987.
14   Davison, G.C., Neale J.M. *Abnormal Psychology: An experimental clinical approach.* Chichester: Wiley, 1986.
15   Reynolds, W., Cormack, D. (eds) *Psychiatric and Mental Health Nursing.* London: Chapman and Hall, 1990.

PART II: LEARNING DISABILITY
1. Difficulties, disabilities and disadvantages

1 Cromer, R.F. *Language and Thought in Normal and Handicapped Children.* Oxford: Basil Blackwood, 1991.
2 Wood, P. *International Classification of Impairments, Disabilities and Handicaps.* Geneva: World Health Organisation, 1981.
3 Oliver, M. *Social Work with Disabled People.* London: Macmillan, 1983.
4 Finkelstein, V., French, S. Towards a psychology of disability. In: Swain J, Finkelstein V, French, S., Oliver, M. (eds) *Disabling Barriers - Enabling Environments.* London: Sage Publications, 1993.
5 Sutcliffe, J. *Adults with Learning Difficulties: Education for choice and empowerment.* Leicester: National Institute of Adult Continuing Education, 1990.
6 Alaszewski, A. From villains to victims. In: Leighton, A. (ed). *Mental Handicap in the Community.* London: Woodhead-Faulkner, 1988.
7 McGill, P., Cummings, R. An analysis of the representation of people with mental handicaps in a British newspaper. *Mental Handicap Research* 1990; 3: 1, 60-69.
8 Kay, A. Helping with social issues. In: Shanley, E., Starrs, T. (eds) *Learning Disabilities: A handbook of care* (second edition). Edinburgh: Churchill Livingstone, 1993.
9 Brown, H., Smith, H. *Normalisation: A model for the nineties.* London: Tavistock/Routledge, 1992.
10 Brechin, A., Swain, J. Creating a 'working alliance' with people with learning difficulties. In: Brechin, A., Walmsley, J. (eds) *Making Connections: Reflecting on the lives and experiences of people with learning difficulties.* London: Hodder and Stoughton, 1989.
11 Alaszewski, A., Ong, B.N. (eds). *Normalisation in Practice: Residential care for children with a profound mental handicap.* London: Routledge, 1990.
12 Jupp, K. *Living a Full Life with Learning Disabilities.* London: Souvenir Press, 1994.
13 Finkelstein, V. Disability and the helper/helped relationship: an historical view. In: Brechin, A., Liddiard, P., Swain, J. (eds) *Handicap in a Social World.* London: Hodder and Stoughton; Milton Keynes: The Open University Press, 1981.

2. Children and families

1 Worsley, P. *Introducing Sociology.* Harmondsworth: Penguin, 1976.
2 Petrie, G. Physical causes and conditions. In: Shanley, E., Starrs, T. (eds) *Learning Disabilities: A handbook of care* (second edition). Edinburgh: Churchill Livingstone, 1993.
3 Sinson, J.C. *Attitudes to Down's Syndrome - An investigation of attitudes to mental handicap in urban and rural Yorkshire.* London: Mental Health Foundation, 1985.
4 Cunningham, C., Davies, H. Parent counselling. In: Craft, M., Bicknell, J., Hollins, S. (eds) *Mental handicap: A multidisciplinary approach.* London: Baillière Tindall, 1985.
5 Worthington, A. *Coming to Terms with Mental Handicap.* Whitby: Helena Press, 1985.
6 Mathias, P. Family vulnerability, support networks and counselling. In: Thompson, T., Mathias, P. (eds) *Standards and Mental Handicap.* London: Baillière Tindall, 1992.
7 Byrne, E.A., Cunningham, C.C., Sloper, P. *Families and Their Children with Down's Syndrome: One feature in common.* London: Routledge, 1988.
8 Glendinning, C. Community care: the financial consequences for women. In: Glendinning, C., Millar, J. (eds) *Women and Poverty in Britain: The 1990s.* London: Harvester Wheatsheaf, 1992.
9 Sutcliffe, J., Simons, K. *Self-advocacy and Adults with Learning Difficulties.* Leicester: National Institute of Adult Continuing Education, 1993.
10 Hall, L. Severe learning difficulties: educational provision. In: Thompson, T., Mathias, P. (eds). *Standards and Mental Handicap.* London: Baillière Tindall, 1992.
11 Byrne, E.A., Cunningham, C.C., Sloper, P. *Families and their Children with Down's Syndrome. One feature in common.* London: Routledge, 1988.
12 MacKay, G. Helping with learning difficulties. In: Shanley, E., Starrs, T. (eds). *Learning Disabilities: A handbook of care* (second edition). Edinburgh: Churchill Livingstone, 1993.

3. Becoming an adult

1 Jenkins, R. Barriers to adulthood: long-term unemployment and mental handicap compared. In: Brechin, A., Walmsley, J. (eds) *Making Connections: Reflecting on the lives and experiences of people with learning difficulties.* London: Hodder and Stoughton, 1989, p.102.

2 Lea, S.J. Mental retardation: social construction or clinical reality? *Disability, Handicap and Society* 1988; 3: 1, 65–66.

3 McConkey, R. Our young lives: school leavers' impressions and those of their parents to life at home and their hopes for the future. In: McConkey, R., Conliffe, C. (eds) *The Person with Mental Handicap: Preparation for an adult life in the community.* Dublin: St. Michael's House; Belfast: Institute of Counselling and Personal Development, 1989, p.32.

4 Ayer, S., Alaszewski, A. *Community Care and the Mentally Handicapped: Services for mothers and their mentally handicapped children.* London: Croom Helm, 1986, p,227.

5 Baxter, C., Poonia, K., Ward, L., Nadirshaw, Z. *Double Discrimination: Issues and services for people with learning difficulties from black and ethnic minority communities.* London: King's Fund Centre, 1990.

6 Crosskill, D., Bano, A. Helping personal and sexual relationships in a multiracial society. In: Thompson, T., Mathias, P. (eds). *Standards and Mental Handicap.* London: Baillière Tindall, 1992.

7 Brearley, P., Mandelstam, M. *A Review of Literature 1986 – 1991 on Day Care Services for Adults.* Prepared by the Disabled Living Foundation for the Social Services Inspectorate. London: HMSO, 1992, p.8.

8 Whittaker, A., Wright, J., Bourlet, G. Setting up for self-advocacy. In: Booth, T. (ed) *Better Lives: Changing services for people with learning difficulties. Social Service monographs: Research in Practice.* Sheffield: Joint Unit for Social Services Research at Sheffield University, 1990, p.80.

9 Carr, J., Collins, S. *Working Towards Independence: A practical guide to teaching people with learning disabilities.* London: Jessica Kingsley, 1992.

10 MacLachlan, M., Dennis, P., Lang, H., Charnock, S., Osman, J. Do the professionals understand? Mothers' views of families' service needs. In: Brechin, A., Walmsley, J. (eds) *Making Connections: Reflecting on the lives and experiences of people with learning difficulties.* London: Hodder and Stoughton, 1989.

11 Hogg, J., Moss, S., Cooke, D. Ageing and mental handicap. Leighton, A. (ed). In: *Mental Handicap in the Community.* London: Woodhead Faulkner, 1988, pp.155-170.

12 Sinson, J.C. *Group Homes and Community Integration of Developmentally Disabled People: Micro-institutionalisation?* London: Jessica Kingsley, 1993.

4. Creating healthy services

1 Royal College of Nursing Community Nursing Forum for People with a Learning Disability. *The Role and Function of the Domiciliary Nurse for People with a Learning Disability.* London: Royal College of Nursing, 1992, p.23.

2 Report of the working group commissioned by the four chief nursing officers of the United Kingdom. *Caring for People: Community care in the next decade and beyond - Mental Handicap Nursing.* (The Cullen Report.) London: Department of Health 1991.

3 Plank, M. *Teams for Mentally Handicapped People.* London: Campaign for Mental Handicap (now Values into Action), 1981.

4 Griffiths, T., Brown, S. *Register of Community Mental Handicap Teams in England.* Centre for Research in Social Policy. Loughborough: Loughborough University of Technology, 1990, p.vi.

5 Mansell, J. The natural history of the community mental handicap team. In: Brown, S., Wistow, G. (eds) *The Roles and Tasks of Community Mental Handicap Teams.* Aldershot: Gower, 1990.

6 Audit Commission for Local Authorities in England and Wales. *Making a Reality of Community Care.* London: HMSO, 1986.

7 HMSO. *Community Care: Agenda for action.* (The Griffiths Report). London: HMSO, 1988.

8 Department of Health, Department of Social Security, Welsh Office and Scottish Office. *Caring for People: Community care in the next decade and beyond.* (White Paper) London: HMSO, 1989. (Cmnd 849.)

9 Sines, D. Service provision: developments in the National Health Service. In: Thompson, T., Mathias, P. (eds). *Standards and Mental Handicap.* London: Baillière Tindall, 1992.

10 Department of Health. *Services for People with Learning Disabilities and Challenging Behaviour or Mental Health Needs.* (The Mansell Report.) London: HMSO, 1993.

11 Department of Health/Home Office. *Review of Health and Social Services for Mentally Disordered Offenders and Others Requiring Similar Services.* Volume 7: *People with learning disabilities (mental handicap) or autism.* London: HMSO, 1994.

12 Collins, J. *When Eagles Fly: A report on the resettlement of people with learning difficulties from long-stay institutions.* London: Values Into Action, 1992.

13 Morris, J. *Community Care or Independent Living?* York: Joseph Rowntree Foundation, 1993.

14 Zarb, G., Nadash, P. *Cashing in on Independence: Comparing the costs and benefits of cash and Services.* Derbyshire: Belper, British Council of Organisations of Disabled People, 1994.

15 Joseph Rowntree Foundation. *Joseph Rowntree Findings. Employing personal assistants. Social Care Research, No 61.* York: Joseph Rowntree Foundation, 1995.